Clinical Focus on Dermatology
SEXUALLY TRANSMITTED INFECTIONS
(Under the Aegis of IADVL WB Academy)

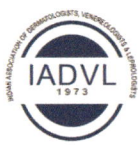

Clinical Focus on Dermatology

SEXUALLY TRANSMITTED INFECTIONS

(Under the Aegis of IADVL WB Academy)

Editor

Sudip Das MD(Dermatology and Venereology) (AIIMS New Delhi) FRCP(Edinburgh)
Professor and Head
Department of Dermatology
Calcutta National Medical College and Hospital
Kolkata, West Bengal, India

Associate Editor

Kingshuk Chatterjee MBBS DNB(DVL) MNAMS IFAAD FAGE
FRCP(Edinburgh, Glasgow, and London)
Associate Professor
Department of Dermatology
Nil Ratan Sircar Medical College
Kolkata, West Bengal, India

Foreword

Murugan Sankaranantham

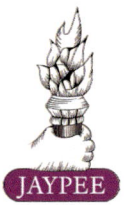

JAYPEE BROTHERS MEDICAL PUBLISHERS
The Health Sciences Publisher
New Delhi | London

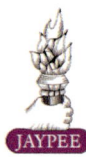

Jaypee Brothers Medical Publishers (P) Ltd

Headquarters
EMCA House, 23/23-B
Ansari Road, Daryaganj
New Delhi 110 002, India
Landline: +91-11-23272143, +91-11-23272703
+91-11-23282021, +91-11-23245672
e-mail: jaypee@jaypeebrothers.com

Corporate Office
4838/24, Ansari Road, Daryaganj
New Delhi 110 002, India
Phone: +91-11-43574357
Fax: +91-11-43574314
e-mail: jaypee@jaypeebrothers.com

Overseas Office
JP Medical Ltd.
83, Victoria Street, London
SW1H 0HW (UK)
Phone: +44-20 3170 8910
e-mail: info@jpmedpub.com

EU GPSR Authorised Representative
Logos Europe, 9 rue Nicolas Poussin
17000, La Rochelle, France
Phone: +33 (0) 6 67 93 73 78
e-mail: contact@logoseurope.eu

Website: www.jaypeebrothers.com
Website: www.jaypeedigital.com

© 2026, Jaypee Brothers Medical Publishers

The views and opinions expressed in this book are solely those of the original contributor(s)/author(s) and do not necessarily represent those of editor(s) or publisher of the book.

All rights reserved. No part of this publication may be reproduced, stored or transmitted in any form or by any means, electronic, mechanical, photocopying, recording or otherwise, without the prior permission in writing of the publishers.

All brand names and product names used in this book are trade names, service marks, trademarks or registered trademarks of their respective owners. The publisher is not associated with any product or vendor mentioned in this book.

Medical knowledge and practice change constantly. This book is designed to provide accurate, authoritative information about the subject matter in question. However, readers are advised to check the most current information available on procedures included and check information from the manufacturer of each product to be administered, to verify the recommended dose, formula, method and duration of administration, adverse effects and contraindications. It is the responsibility of the practitioner to take all appropriate safety precautions. Neither the publisher nor the author(s)/editor(s) assume any liability for any injury and/or damage to persons or property arising from or related to use of material in this book.

This book is sold on the understanding that the publisher is not engaged in providing professional medical services. If such advice or services are required, the services of a competent medical professional should be sought.

Every effort has been made where necessary to contact holders of copyright to obtain permission to reproduce copyright material. If any have been inadvertently overlooked, the publisher will be pleased to make the necessary arrangements at the first opportunity.

Inquiries for bulk sales may be solicited at: jaypee@jaypeebrothers.com

Clinical Focus on Dermatology: Sexually Transmitted Infections / Sudip Das, Kingshuk Chatterjee

First Edition: **2026**
ISBN: 978-93-7202-687-0
Printed in India

Contributors

Abheek Sil MD DNB SCE MNAMS
Assistant Professor
Department of Dermatology, Venereology and Leprosy
PKG Medical College and Hospital
Kolkata, West Bengal, India

Anupam Das MBBS(Hons) MD(Dermatology) (Gold Medalist)
Assistant Professor
Department of Dermatology
KPC Medical College
Kolkata, West Bengal, India

Apeksha Singh MBBS DVDL DNB
Senior Resident
Department of Dermatology
Calcutta National Medical College and Hospital
Kolkata, West Bengal, India

Deepika Pandhi MD FAMS
Senior Resident
Department of Dermatology
University College of Medical Sciences and GTB Hospital
New Delhi, India

Farhat Fatima MBBS MD MRCP SCE
Senior Resident
Department of Dermatology
Calcutta National Medical College and Hospital
Kolkata, West Bengal, India

Indrashis Podder MD DNB MNAMS
Assistant Professor
Department of Dermatology
College of Medicine and Sagore Dutta Hospital
Kolkata, West Bengal, India

Kingshuk Chatterjee MBBS DNB(DVL) MNAMS IFAAD FAGE FRCP(Edinburgh, Glasgow, and London)
Associate Professor
Department of Dermatology
Nil Ratan Sircar Medical College
Kolkata, West Bengal, India

Konakanchi Venkata Chalam MD DVL
Professor
Department of Dermatology, Venereology, and Leprosy
Government Medical College
Srikakulam, Andhra Pradesh, India

Loknath Ghoshal MD
Dermatologist
Department of Dermatology
Nil Ratan Sircar Medical College
Kolkata, West Bengal, India

Padmasri Somala Y MD DVL
Assistant Professor
Department of Dermatology
Government Medical College
Vizianagram, Andhra Pradesh, India

Satarupa Kumar MBBS(Hons) MD(DVL) SCE(UK) Dermatology PGDMLE(NLSIU)
Consultant Dermatologist
Wizderm Speciality Skin and Hair Clinic, Jodhpur Park
Kolkata, West Bengal, India

SK Shahriar Ahmed MBBS MD DNB
Senior Resident
Department of Dermatology
Calcutta National Medical College and Hospital
Kolkata, West Bengal, India

Suchibrata Das MD
Associate Professor
Nil Ratan Sircar Medical College
Kolkata, West Bengal, India

Sudip Das MD(Dermatology and Venereology) (AIIMS New Delhi) FRCP(Edinburgh)
Professor and Head
Department of Dermatology
Calcutta National Medical College and Hospital
Kolkata, West Bengal, India

Vishal Pal MD
Director Professor
Department of Dermatology
University College of Medical Sciences and GTB Hospital
New Delhi, India

Yashpal Manchanda MD
Consultant, Dermatology
PGE Office, Kuwait Institute for Medical Specialization, Sulaibikhat, Jamal Abdul-Nasser Street, Kuwait

Foreword

As long as the human race remains sexually active, sexually transmitted infections (STIs) will also be there. Due to the enormous changes in lifestyle activities such as men having sex with men (MSM), proliferation of massage parlors, weekend parties, usage of abusive drugs, vast migration of people, living-together cultures, dating apps for MSM and for seeking heterosexual partners, influence of social media, etc., there is an upsurge in STIs all over the world.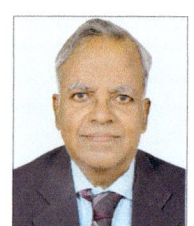

In such situations, our young dermatovenerelogists lose interest in the subject of STIs and their attention diverts toward cosmetology, aesthetics, and dermatosurgical modalities. There are not many recent and more authenticated books exclusively for STIs.

At this juncture, the effort to bring out an interesting and wonderful book on STIs is to be appreciated extravagantly. I congratulate Dr Sudip Das and his team for bringing out a wonderful and handy book on STIs with the recent advances that will be extremely beneficial for the young budding dermatovenereologists as ready reckoner.

The topics are selected nicely and covered. The authors described the lesions with nice clinical pictures and tables. The editors not only described the clinical presentations and management aspects, but also covered nicely the preventive measures and vaccines and touched on the aspect of recent advances in the field of STI/HIV. This book must be in the hands of every postgraduate in the field of dermatovenereology, and adequate copies should also be made available in the college libraries of all teaching institutions across the country.

Murugan Sankaranantham
Senior Consultant in STI/HIV and Sexual Medicine
SHIFA Hospitals, Tirunelveli, Tamil Nadu, India
Former Professor and Head
Department of Dermatology, Venereology and Leprosy
Sree Mookambika Institute of Medical Sciences
Kulasekaram, Kanyakumari District, Tamil Nadu, India
Past National President, Indian Association for the Study of
Sexually Transmitted Diseases and AIDS (IASSTD and AIDS)

Preface

Sexually transmitted infections (STIs) continue to be a significant public health challenge worldwide, with profound implications for individual health, reproductive outcomes, and societal well-being. Dermatologists, particularly those trained in venereology, play a pivotal role in the identification, management, and prevention of these infections, given the frequent cutaneous and mucosal manifestations.

This textbook *"Clinical Focus on Dermatology: Sexually Transmitted Infections"* has been conceived as a comprehensive and clinically oriented resource to support postgraduate students, academicians, and practicing clinicians in mastering the diagnosis and management of STIs. The content encompasses classical presentations as well as emerging trends, including antimicrobial resistance, HIV co-infection, viral STIs, and syndromic management approaches, all within the framework of evidence-based medicine and public health guidelines.

The book is structured to facilitate easy learning and retention, with chapters covering clinical features, diagnostic algorithms, treatment protocols, patient counseling, and legal and ethical considerations. Special emphasis has been placed on integrating recent advances in molecular diagnostics, vaccine updates, sexual health education, and the evolving epidemiology of STIs in the postpandemic era.

This effort is the culmination of insights from leading experts in dermatology, venereology, microbiology, and infectious diseases, along with inputs from frontline clinicians who bring the perspective of ground realities. It is our hope that this book not only aids in examination preparedness but also strengthens clinical acumen, fosters empathy, and promotes responsible sexual health practices.

We dedicate this textbook to all learners and caregivers striving to combat the stigma, complications, and transmission of STIs and to make sexual health a priority in comprehensive patient care.

Sudip Das
Kingshuk Chatterjee

Acknowledgments

The work done in this book *"Clinical Focus on Dermatology: Sexually Transmitted Infections"* has ultimately come to fruition through the efforts, ideas, thoughts, dedication, and invaluable time of many faculties and residents, whom I acknowledge from the core of my heart.

I extend my sincere thanks to the then president of IADVL WB, Dr Kaushik Lahiri, who helped us in bringing this book to light. The whole IADVL EC (Executive Committee) helped us in making this dream come true.

I am also indebted to my colleagues, my seniors, and my residents for making this collective effort successful and worthy. I am grateful to the team of Jaypee Brothers Medical Publishers, comprising Mr Ankit Vij (Managing Director), Sabyasachi Hazra (Director, PG & PNR Content), and Akhilesh Saxena (Development Editor), for the tremendous efforts for bringing out this book.

Blessings from the Almighty!

Sudip Das

Contents

CHAPTER 1: **Introduction to Sexually Transmitted Infections**   1
Loknath Ghoshal, Kingshuk Chatterjee

CHAPTER 2: **Genital Ulcer Disease**   8
Sudip Das, SK Shahriar Ahmed

CHAPTER 3: **Discharge**   14
Sudip Das, Apeksha Singh

CHAPTER 4: **Anogenital Warts**   24
Konakanchi Venkata Chalam, Padmasri Somala Y

CHAPTER 5: **Cutaneous Manifestations of HIV**   33
Suchibrata Das, Kingshuk Chatterjee

CHAPTER 6: **Danger of Men Who have Sex with Men, Newer Sexually Transmitted Infections, and Sexual Abuse**   47
Vishal Pal, Deepika Pandhi

CHAPTER 7: **Genital Vaccines**   55
Farhat Fatima, Satarupa Kumar, Anupam Das

CHAPTER 8: **Sexually Transmitted Infection Control Programs**   65
Abheek Sil, Indrashis Podder

CHAPTER 9: **Recent Advances in Management of Sexually Transmitted Diseases**   82
Yashpal Manchanda, Sudip Das

Index   91

CHAPTER 1

Introduction to Sexually Transmitted Infections

Loknath Ghoshal, Kingshuk Chatterjee

INTRODUCTION

Sexually transmitted diseases (STDs) have afflicted humanity for centuries. Prior to the advent of modern medicine, the absence of awareness and effective treatment options contributed to the widespread transmission of these infections. Historically, syphilis and gonorrhea were among the most commonly reported STDs in medieval Europe. One theory posits that syphilis was brought to Europe by crew members of Christopher Columbus, who may have contracted the infection during their expeditions in the Americas and transmitted it upon returning to European ports. Similarly, sailors during Captain Cook's voyages are believed to have introduced gonorrhea to New Zealand from Tahiti.[1]

Sexually transmitted infections (STIs) involve the transmission of an organism between sexual partners through different routes of sexual contact, either oral, anal, or vaginal. A STD develops because of an STI, and the term implies that the infection has led to some symptom(s) of a disease. Often these two terms are used interchangeably. Since the primary goal of public health is prevention and treatment of infections before they develop into a disease, the term STI is more prudent in the context of modern medicine. The most common STIs include both curable (gonorrhea, chlamydia, syphilis, and trichomonas) and treatable [herpes viruses, human papillomavirus (HPV), and human immunodeficiency virus (HIV)] infections. The correlating symptoms are generally classified into two categories—(1) discharge/dysuria and (2) ulcerative lesions.[2]

EPIDEMIOLOGY

Sexually transmitted infections have an intense impact on sexual and reproductive health worldwide. The following data may be useful to comprehend the burden implied. The World Health Organization (WHO) estimates more than a million STIs to be acquired daily, throughout the world.[3] The infections mostly are asymptomatic. Also, every year 374 million persons acquire a new infection with one of four curable STIs (chlamydia, trichomoniasis, gonorrhea, and syphilis).[4] Of these, trichomoniasis is the most common, with 156 million new cases, followed by chlamydia (127 million), gonorrhea (87 million), and syphilis (6.3 million) yearly **(Fig. 1)**.

More than 500 million people in the age group of 15–49 years are estimated to have genital infection with herpes simplex virus (HSV).[5]

Over 311,000 cervical cancer deaths occur each year and is associated with the presence

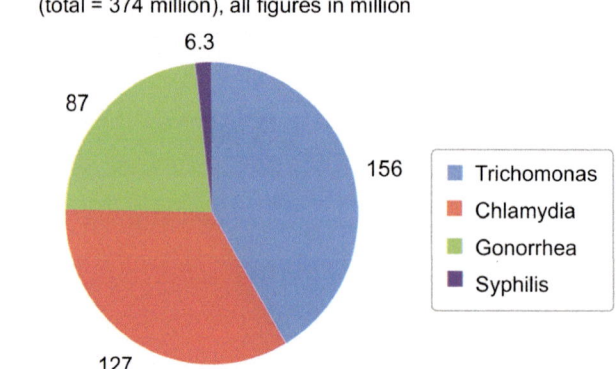

FIG. 1: Incidence of sexually transmitted infection (STI) episodes worldwide.

of HPV infection.[6] HPV is also the cause of anal cancer among men who have sex with men (MSM).

In 2016, nearly 1 million pregnant women were infected with syphilis and resulted in >350,000 adverse birth outcomes.[7] Also, an estimated 296 million people are living with chronic hepatitis B globally. Over and above, STIs have a direct impact on sexual and reproductive health by means of stigmatization, infertility, cancers, and pregnancy-related complications. Also, it is directly implicated in acquiring HIV infection, multiplying the chance of sexual acquisition to almost 10-fold. The problem of worldwide drug resistance is a major blockage in the control of STIs.

The Centre for Disease Control and Prevention (CDC) reported a gradual decrease in syphilis, gonorrhea, and chancroid over the years except in the case of chlamydial infection (1,307,893 cases in 2010).[8]

There was increase in new cases of chlamydia, gonorrhea, trichomoniasis, and genital herpes between 1990 and 2013. Peak ages for new infection in each STI were between 20 and 25 years and largely remained constant from 1990 to 2013. According to global estimates, the most common acute STI in females is trichomoniasis and chlamydia in males. Genital herpes seemed to be the most common chronic infection in both males and females.[9]

INDIAN SCENARIO

There is lack of community based and comprehensive surveillance system in this regard and thus, the exact extent of the problem remains unknown. A community-based survey by Indian Council of Medical Research (ICMR) in 2002–2003 showed that 5–6% sexually active adult population suffer from STIs [rapid assessment survey (RAS) 2005]. The 2005 ICMR multicenter RAS indicates that 12% of female clients and 6% of male clients attending the outpatient departments seek advice related to STIs [The National Family Health Survey (NFHS-3)]. Still, the level of awareness and treatment seeking behavior remains low in India despite the high incidence of STIs (Behavioural Surveillance Survey (BSS 2006)].[10]

There is a marked diversity in the recorded epidemiology of different STIs/reproductive tract infections (RTIs) in the country (mid-term report 2010) diverse.[11] STDs and HIV are the main causes of lost healthy lives in 15–40 years males (almost 15%). It is interesting that the rate of STI/RTI in rural and urban areas is the same. This implicates that the factors leading to acquisition of STI/RTI are the same in both the areas. It is possibly the recent rapid urbanization that is responsible for the similarity in this regard.

In India, around 6% of the adult population has one or more STI/RTI which totals to the occurrence of about 30–35 million episodes of STI/RTI every year. The prevalence of STI/RTI in the general population based on various data after the year 2020 gives no definite trend **(Table 1)**.

The HIV prevalence—there are approximately 2.4 million people in India living with HIV in India implying an adult prevalence of 0.3%. The prevalence of HIV is extraordinary in the 15–49 age groups and makes for 88.7% of all infections. More males are HIV positive than females. The prevalence rate for adult females is 0.29 %, while for males it is 0.43% when accounted overall. In India, there are 195 high priority districts of which 156 are considered category A districts [>1% antenatal clinic (ANC) prevalence] and 39 are designated as category B districts (<1% ANC prevalence and > 5% prevalence in any high-risk group site). The mode of transmission of STI and HIV is same; presence of STI enhances the HIV acquisition and transmission risk by upto 10 times.[12,13]

CLASSIFICATION

Sexually transmitted infections can either be classified according to causative pathogens/treatment response **(Table 2)**.

If we consider disease wise, STIs can also be classified as:
- *Curable*:
    - Syphilis
    - Gonorrhea
    - Lymphogranuloma venereum
    - Chancroid
- *Treatable*:
    - HHV (human herpesvirus) infection
    - HIV infection[15]

CONTROL OF SEXUALLY TRANSMITTED INFECTION

The WHO recognizes, as part of global health strategies the significance of controlling STIs and RTIs. The WHO highlights four key elements for STI control—case reporting, prevalence assessment, etiologies, and monitoring antimicrobial resistance.[16] Global control and prevention of STIs contribute to achieving universal access to sexual and reproductive healthcare services and align with sustainable development goals.

Strategies of STI/RTI prevention and control include (1) provision of standardized STI/RTI management to general population, (2) provision of standardized STI/RTI management to high-risk group population, and (3) provision of laboratory surveillance of STI/RTI.

At the national level, the National AIDS Control Programme (NACP) was launched in 1987. As national response to contain the HIV epidemic, Government of India set up the National AIDS Control Organization (NACO), a separate wing to monitor the implementation of NACP. The program is

TABLE 1: Prevalence of STI in males and females.

STI	Female (%)	Male (%)
Genital discharge	8–51	0.2–6.6
Genital ulcer disease	0–7.8	0.7–2
Lower abdominal pain	0.6–37	–
Scrotal swelling	–	0–1.5
Inguinal swelling	–	0.3–1.7
Syphilis	0–4.7	1–16.1
Gonorrhea	0–1.9	0–3.9
Chlamydia	0–1.3	0–1.1
Trichomonas vaginalis	1.2–8	1.5–3.6
Candidiasis	7.2–23.9	–
Bacterial vaginosis	17.8–63.7	–
Herpes simplex virus 2	8.6–17.9	7–10.6
HIV	0–0.95	0–1.4

(STI: sexually transmitted infection; HIV: human immunodeficiency viruses)

TABLE 2: Etiological classification of STIs.

Pathogen	Infection
Parasites	*Trichomonas vaginalis, Sarcoptes scabiei,* and *Phthirus pubis*
Fungi	Trichophyton mentagrophytes subspecies *Note: Candida albicans* is only facultatively pathogenic and does not cause STIs
Bacteria	*Chlamydia trachomatis* (serotypes D-K and serotypes L1-L3), *Klebsiella granulomatosis, Neisseria gonorrhoeae, Treponema pallidum, Haemophilus ducreyi;* and *Mycoplasma genitalium*
Viruses	Human papillomaviruses, herpes simplex virus, HIV, hepatitis B virus, hepatitis C virus, molluscum contagiosum virus, and monkeypox virus[14]

(HIV: human immunodeficiency virus; STI: sexually transmitted infection)

TABLE 3: Important historical landmarks of NACO.

Year	Milestone achieved
1992	National AIDS Control Programme (NACP-I) was launched to slow the spread of HIV infection. National AIDS Control Board was constituted and NACO was set up
1999	NACP-II began; stressed on behavior change, increased decentralization, and increasing NGO involvement. SACS were established
2007	NACP-III launched for 5 years (2007–2012)
2014	NACP-IV launched for 5 years (2012–2017)

(AIDS: acquired immunodeficiency syndrome; HIV: human immunodeficiency virus; NACO: National AIDS Control Organization; SACS: State AIDS Prevention and Control Societies)

implemented at the state level by the State AIDS Prevention and Control Societies (SACS) **(Table 3)**. The basic milestones in this regard are given in **Table 3**.

Classification of states and districts based on HIV prevalence—based on sentinel surveillance data, the states can be classified into group 1 (high prevalence states, group 2 (moderate prevalence) and group 3 (low prevalence states). Also, the districts have been classified according to last 3 years data into categories A, B, C, and D in decreasing ANC and parent-to-child transmission (PTCT) service prevalence.

Sexually Transmitted Infection Control Program

The STD control is closely linked to HIV/acquired immunodeficiency syndrome (AIDS) control as behavior resulting in the transmission of STD and HIV is similar. HIV is transmissible more easily in the presence of another STD. Hence, early diagnosis and treatment of STD is now recognized as one of the major strategies to control spread of HIV infection.

It was additionally decided to unify services for the treatment of RTIs and STIs across all levels of healthcare. STI clinics at the district/block/first referral unit (FRU) level serve as referral centers for the treatment of STIs referred from the periphery. STI clinics in all district hospitals, medical colleges, and other facilities are strengthened with technical assistance, equipment, reagents, and drugs. A massive orientation-training program was implemented to instruct all medical and paramedical staff involved in providing STD/RTI services using a syndromic approach. All STI clinics offer counseling services and high-quality condoms to STI patients. NGOs' services are also used to provide such counseling services at STI clinics. NACO has named the STI/RTI services as "Suraksha Clinic" and has developed a communication strategy for generation of demand for these services. Prepacked color-coded STI/RTI kits have been provided for free supply to all designated STI/RTI clinics for syndromic management (management of STDs based on specific symptoms and signs and not dependent on laboratory investigations) **(Table 4)**.[17] These kits are color coded are given here.

Counseling and HIV Testing Services

The HIV counseling and testing services include the components as (1) Integrated Counseling and Testing Centres (ICTC), (2) prevention of parent-to-child transmission of HIV (PPTCT), and (3) HIV/tuberculosis collaborative activities. ICTC may be either fixed or mobile centers **(Box 1)**. The fixed facility centers may also be standalone ICTC (SA-ICTC) or facility integrated (F-ICTC).[17]

TABLE 4: Kits for syndromic management of sexually transmitted infection.

Kit no.	Color	Composition	Indication
1.	Gray	Tablet azithromycin 1 g + tablet cefixime 800 mg single dose	• Urethral discharge syndrome • Vaginal discharge syndrome (cervicitis) • Painful scrotal swelling • Presumptive treatment (PT)
2.	Green	Tablet secnidazole 2 g + tablet fluconazole 150 mg single dose	Vaginal discharge syndrome (vaginitis)
3.	White	• Injection benzathine penicillin G 2.4 MU and tablet azithromycin 1 g single dose • 10 mL disposable syringe with 21 G needle and 10 mL of sterile water	Genital ulcer disease syndrome (for syphilis and chancroid)
4.	Blue	Tablet doxycycline 100 mg (28 capsules as twice daily for 14 days) + tablet azithromycin 1 g single dose	Genital ulcer disease syndrome (for syphilis and chancroid during unavailability or history of allergy to BPG)
5.	Red	Tablet acyclovir 400 mg (21 tablets as thrice daily dose for 21 days)	Genital ulcer disease syndrome (for herpetic ulcer)
6.	Yellow	Tablet cefixime 800 mg single dose + tablet metronidazole 400 mg (28 tablets as twice daily for 14 days) + capsule doxycycline 100 mg (28 capsules as twice daily for 14 days)	• Lower abdominal pain • Pelvic inflammatory disease
7.	Black	Tablet doxycycline 100 mg (42 capsules as twice daily for 21 days)	• Inguinal bubo under genital ulcer disease syndrome • Lymphogranuloma venereum (LGV) proctitis under anorectal discharge syndrome
8.	Brown	Tablet cefixime 800 mg single dose + tablet doxycycline 100 mg (14 capsules as twice daily for 7 days)	Anorectal discharge syndrome

> **BOX 1: Basic principles of STI control program.**
> - Meeting STI/RTI needs of general population and bridge population through designated STI/RTI clinics at district hospitals and teaching hospitals attached to medical colleges
> - Subdistrict level health facilities [primary health centers (PHC) and community health centers (CHC)]
> - STI/RTI services to high-risk groups (HRG) by ensuring provision of essential STI service package (ESP) through specified clinic settings involving preferred private providers
> - Treatment of STI using syndromic approach and standardized STI treatment in the form of prepackaged drug kits
> - Counseling through a dedicated counselor at the designated clinics
> - Demand generation for STI/RTI services through branding as "Suraksha Clinic", and mass and mid-media activities including RRC and radio campaigns
> - Strengthening of Regional STI Training Research and Reference Laboratories (RSTRRL)
>
> (RTI: reproductive tract infection; RRC: Red Ribbon Club; STI: sexually transmitted infection)

CONCLUSION

Sexually transmitted infections lead to significant morbidity and mortality across different age groups of the population. Changing socio-economic pattern and sexual orientation contributes significantly toward challenges faced during diagnosis and management of such infections. Adequate knowledge about pathogenesis and government initiated control programmes will only help us to bring down the STI burden.

REFERENCES

1. Burg G. History of sexually transmitted infections (STI). G Ital Dermatol Venereol. 2012;147(4):329-40.
2. CDC: Centers for Disease Control and Prevention. (2024). Sexually Transmitted Infections (STIs). [online] Available from https://www.cdc.gov/sti/about/index.html [Last accessed June, 2025].
3. Tuddenham S, Hamill MM, Ghanem KG. Diagnosis and Treatment of Sexually Transmitted Infections: A Review. JAMA. 2022;327:161-72.
4. World Health Organization. (2022). Sexually Transmitted Infections (STIs). [online] Available from https://www.who.int/news-room/fact-sheets/detail/sexually-transmitted-infections-(stis) [Last accessed June, 2025].
5. James C, Harfouche M, Welton NJ, Turner KM, Abu-Raddad LJ, Gottlieb SL, et al. Herpes simplex virus: Global infection prevalence and incidence estimates, 2016. Bull World Health Organ. 2020;98(5):315-29.
6. Bray F, Ferlay J, Soerjomataram I, Siegel RL, Torre LA, Jemal A. Global cancer statistics 2018: GLOBOCAN estimates of incidence and mortality worldwide for 36 cancers in 185 countries. CA Cancer J Clin. 2018;68(6):394-424.
7. Unemo M, Lahra MM, Escher M, Eremin S, Cole MJ, Galarza P, et al. WHO global antimicrobial resistance surveillance (GASP/GLASS) for *Neisseria gonorrhoeae* 2017-2018: a retrospective observational study. Lancet Microbe. 2021;2:e627-36.
8. Workowski KA, Bolan GA; Centers for Disease Control and Prevention. Sexually transmitted diseases treatment guidelines, 2015. MMWR Recomm Rep. 2015;64(RR-03):1-137.
9. Zheng Y, Yu Q, Lin Y, Zhou Y, Lan L, Yang S, et al. Global burden and trends of sexually transmitted infections from 1990 to 2019: an observational trend study. Lancet Infect Dis. 2022;22(4):541-551.
10. Prabha ML, Sasikala G, Bala S. Comparison of syndromic diagnosis of reproductive tract infections with laboratory diagnosis among rural married women in Medak district, Andhra Pradesh. Indian J Sex Transm Dis AIDS. 2012;33(2):112-5.

11. National guidelines on prevention treatment and control of STI/RTI. NACO; August 2007. Available from: https://naco.gov.in/sites/default/files/National_Guidelines_on_PMC_of_RTI_Including_STI 1.pdf [Last accessed on July, 2025].
12. National guidelines on prevention treatment and control of STI/RTI. NACO; August 2007.
13. National STI/RTI Control and Prevention Programme. NACP, Phase-III, India. Avaliable at www.nacoonline.org [Last accessed June, 2025].
14. Wihlfahrt K, Günther V, Mendling W, Westermann A, Willer D, Gitas G, et al. Sexually Transmitted Diseases-An Update and Overview of Current Research. Diagnostics (Basel). 2023;13(9):1656.
15. Garcia MR, Leslie SW, Wray AA. Sexually Transmitted Infections. In: StatPearls. Treasure Island (FL): StatPearls Publishing; 2025.
16. WHO. (2005). Sexually Transmitted and Other Reproductive Tract Infections. A guide to essential practice. [online] Available from https://iris.who.int/bitstream/handle/10665/43116/9241592656.pdf;jsessionid=765731114C58E108F1C2215DD2C3F576?sequence=1 [Last accessed June, 2025].
17. Strategy Document. National AIDS and STD Control Programme Phase-V (2021-2026). [online] Available from https://naco.gov.in/sites/default/files [Last accessed June, 2025].

CHAPTER 2

Genital Ulcer Disease

Sudip Das, SK Shahriar Ahmed

INTRODUCTION

The prevalence of causative organisms for genital ulcer disease (GUD) varies significantly worldwide and can change over time. Currently, herpes simplex viruses 1 and 2 (HSV-1 and HSV-2) are the most common causes, followed by *Treponema pallidum* (syphilis), *Chlamydia trachomatis* serovars L1–L3 [lymphogranuloma venereum (LGV)], and, less frequently, *Haemophilus ducreyi* (chancroid).[1]

Genital ulcers in primary syphilis often appear before serological tests become positive, making early diagnosis difficult. In areas with high syphilis prevalence, positive serology may reflect a previous, treated infection, even if the current ulcer is due to HSV-2. Clinical diagnosis alone is unreliable, with accuracy rates below 50%, even among experienced clinicians. Therefore, effective GUD management requires either laboratory-based diagnosis or a syndromic approach. Periodic local evaluations of prevalent organisms should guide this approach, ensuring accurate and timely treatment based on the current epidemiological landscape. This strategy helps mitigate misdiagnosis and improves patient outcomes.

GENITAL HERPES

Genital herpes typically presents as clusters of vesicular or ulcerative lesions on the genital or perianal area, but similar appearances may occur with other conditions such as syphilis or chancroid, and these presentations can be further modified by human immunodeficiency virus (HIV) coinfection.[2] First-episode genital herpes, seen in individuals without a previous history, often involves systemic symptoms such as fever, headache, malaise, and myalgia, along with localized pain, itching, dysuria, and tender inguinal lymphadenopathy. Lesions usually begin as papules or vesicles that spread over the genital area, lasting up to 15–20 days until crusting and healing, although crusting does not occur on mucosal surfaces. Primary genital herpes affects seronegative individuals within 5–14 days of exposure, while initial episodes in those with pre-existing HSV-2 antibodies indicate past asymptomatic infections. Recurrent episodes are generally milder, with localized itching and ulcers, lasting about 4–15 days. Examination findings include vesiculopustular or ulcerative lesions on the external genitalia, perianal area, or buttocks, often coalescing into larger ulcers. Many patients present later in the ulcerative stage, lacking the typical vesicular phase, but a history of recurrent ulcers supports a presumptive diagnosis. Immunosuppressed individuals may develop persistent, expanding ulcers that rarely scar due to their shallow intraepidermal nature.[3] Molecular testing, particularly polymerase chain reaction (PCR) of HSV DNA from lesion swabs, is the most sensitive diagnostic method and can also detect *T. pallidum* when combined assays are available. Culture methods, though less commonly used, help confirm diagnoses and assess antiviral resistance, with the highest yield from vesicular lesions. Serology, including type-specific IgG tests for HSV-1 and HSV-2, has limited diagnostic value, primarily useful for detecting seroconversion between the acute phase and 6-12 weeks later. IgM testing is unreliable for identifying new infections, as it can also be present during recurrent episodes, reducing its diagnostic utility.[4]

SYPHILIS

Syphilis, a systemic disease caused by the spirochaete *T. pallidum*, is classified as congenital or acquired. Congenital syphilis is transmitted in utero, while acquired syphilis progresses through early and late stages. Early syphilis includes primary, secondary, and early latent phases (<2 years postinfection), whereas late syphilis encompasses late latent stages, and forms affecting the nervous system, cardiovascular system, and gummatous disease. Primary syphilis typically presents as a single painless chancre at the infection site, developing after an incubation of 9-90 days, which heals within 2-10 weeks if untreated.[5] Secondary syphilis, occurring 6 weeks to 6 months postinfection, is marked by systemic symptoms such as fever, malaise, and arthralgia, along with generalized maculopapular rashes (including palms and soles), patchy alopecia, lymphadenopathy, condylomata lata, and highly contagious mucous membrane ulcers. This stage is often accompanied by a visible chancre, especially in immunosuppressed individuals. If untreated, the disease enters a latent phase, which can be early (<2 years) or late (>2 years). Early latent syphilis is infectious and may relapse into secondary manifestations, while late latent syphilis shows no clinical symptoms and has reduced infectiousness. Diagnostic methods include dark-field microscopy, PCR for *T. pallidum*, and serology. In primary syphilis, serological tests such as rapid plasma reagin (RPR) (nontreponemal) and *T. pallidum* hemagglutination assay (TPHA) (treponemal) may be negative initially but become reactive 1-4 weeks postchancre. Secondary syphilis almost always shows reactive serology, with high nontreponemal titers (≥1:16), though rare false negatives can occur due to the prozone phenomenon. Nontreponemal tests monitor treatment response, as titers decline after effective therapy. Early latent syphilis requires serological confirmation, with reactive nontreponemal and treponemal tests. In late latent syphilis, treponemal tests remain positive for life, while nontreponemal tests may turn negative. Rapid syphilis test functions such as treponemal assays, indicating past exposure but not active infection, and are best paired with RPR to confirm active disease. Serological tests must be interpreted alongside sexual history, physical examination, and recent antibiotic use, as false positives can result from acute illnesses, immunizations, pregnancy, or autoimmune disorders.[6] In high-prevalence areas, repeated serological testing helps avoid unnecessary treatments by distinguishing active from past infections.

CHANCROID

Chancroid, caused by *H. ducreyi*, presents initially as an erythematous papule appearing within hours to days after sexual contact.[7] This papule evolves into a pustule within 1-2 days, eventually breaking down to form a painful ulcer, which typically prompts patients to seek medical care. In men, ulcers commonly occur on the foreskin, penile shaft, or glans, often accompanied by painful unilateral or bilateral inguinal lymphadenopathy. These swollen lymph nodes, or buboes, can become large, fluctuant, and may suppurate, forming fistulae or additional ulcers if untreated. Women generally develop ulcers on the vulva, with potential autoinoculation causing anal lesions. Female chancroid ulcers may be asymptomatic, especially if internal, and women less frequently experience inguinal adenopathy due to differing lymphatic drainage. Clinically, chancroid ulcers are usually deep, with irregular edges and a red margin, often tender during examination or when walking. The base tends to be granular or purulent, with no characteristic induration. However, the presentation can vary; small ulcers might mimic genital herpes, while in HIV-positive or immunosuppressed patients, ulcers can be less purulent, resemble syphilitic chancres, or become rapidly aggressive and erosive, potentially causing extensive genital destruction. Diagnosis of *H. ducreyi* traditionally relied on culture methods, which are limited to specialized centers due to the organism's fastidious nature, yielding about 75% sensitivity compared to multiplex PCR (M-PCR) from genital ulcer swabs. While M-PCR for GUD exists, it remains primarily in research or reference centers.[8] Given the global decline in chancroid cases, further diagnostic advancements are unlikely. Clinicians should maintain a high suspicion for chancroid when encountering painful, suppurative genital ulcers, particularly with inguinal lymphadenopathy in men. Recognizing atypical or unusually aggressive presentations in immunosuppressed individuals is crucial. If a rise in such cases occurs, national health authorities should be notified to adapt treatment protocols accordingly.

LYMPHOGRANULOMA VENEREUM

Lymphogranuloma venereum is a sexually transmitted infection caused by the bacterium *C. trachomatis*, specifically serovars L1, L2, and L3. It is prevalent in tropical and subtropical regions and has seen a resurgence among men who have sex with men, particularly those co-infected with HIV.[9] The infection progresses through three stages:
1. *Primary stage*: It is characterized by painless genital ulcers or papules at the site of inoculation.
2. *Secondary stage*: It is marked by tender inguinal or femoral lymphadenopathy, commonly referred to as buboes.
3. *Tertiary stage*: It involves chronic inflammatory responses leading to fibrosis, strictures, and fistulas in the anogenital region.

Diagnosis is often clinical but can be confirmed through nucleic acid amplification tests (NAATs) detecting *C. trachomatis* DNA. Serological tests may also assist in diagnosis. The recommended treatment is a 21-day course of doxycycline. An alternate regimen is erythromycin 500 mg orally four times a day given for 21 days or azithromycin 1 g orally once weekly for 3 weeks. Early diagnosis and treatment are crucial to prevent complications and transmission. Complications usually occur when the disease is left untreated— necrosis and rupture of the lymph nodes, anogenital fibrosis, strictures, anal fistulae, and elephantiasis. Public health measures, including education and regular screening of high-risk populations, are essential for controlling the spread of LGV.

DONOVANOSIS

Donovanosis, also known as granuloma inguinale, is a chronic, progressive bacterial infection of the genital and perigenital regions caused by *Klebsiella granulomatis*. It is characterized by painless, slowly progressive ulcerative lesions on the genitals or perineum without regional lymphadenopathy. The disease is primarily transmitted through sexual contact, with an incubation period ranging from 1 to

12 weeks. It is more prevalent in tropical and subtropical regions, including India, Papua New Guinea, the Caribbean, South America, and parts of southern Africa. Clinically, donovanosis presents as painless, beefy-red ulcers that bleed easily upon contact. The other types are hypertrophic or verrucous, necrotic, and sclerotic. Without treatment, these lesions can lead to significant tissue destruction and scarring. Diagnosis is confirmed by identifying Donovan bodies—intracellular inclusions within mononuclear phagocytes—in tissue samples stained with Wright–Giemsa or Leishman stains. The recommended treatment duration is a minimum 3-week or until resolution of symptoms. First-line treatment is azithromycin 1 g followed by 500 mg daily. Patients that are slow to respond can also be given gentamicin 500 mg every 8 hours. Erythromycin is the medication of choice in pregnancy. Alternative treatments include doxycycline, ciprofloxacin, or trimethoprim-sulfamethoxazole. Surgery may be needed for extensive tissue destruction. Early diagnosis and complete treatment are essential to prevent complications and reduce transmission. Public health measures, including education, improved access to healthcare, and regular screening of high-risk populations, are crucial for controlling the spread of donovanosis. In regions where the disease is endemic, these strategies have led to a significant decline in incidence.[10]

TREATMENT

For individuals presenting with genital ulcers, including anorectal ulcers, the World Health Organization (WHO) recommends treatment based on quality-assured molecular assays, such as NAAT, to confirm or exclude HSV, *T. pallidum* (syphilis), or LGV if cases are emerging in the region. In settings without molecular tests or laboratory capacity, WHO advises syndromic treatment, ensuring patients receive treatment on the same day. Key practices include taking a thorough medical and sexual history, performing physical examinations of the genital and anal areas, offering HIV and syphilis testing, providing preventive services, and offering analgesics for pain relief. For people with confirmed anogenital ulcers, molecular assays should be performed to confirm or exclude HSV and syphilis and to detect LGV, especially in areas where it is reported. Treatment for syphilis and HSV should follow the results available the same day or syndromically if molecular testing is not available. If LGV is confirmed, treatment should be provided, and chancroid should only be treated in regions where it is endemic. In the absence of molecular testing, treatment should be syndromic, focusing on HSV for recurrent or vesicular ulcers and syphilis for individuals without recent treatment history. Good practice includes serological testing for syphilis, monitoring treatment responses, and referring men with persistent ulcers to specialized centers with diagnostic capacity for HSV and other less common pathogens such as LGV, donovanosis, and chancroid.

For individuals experiencing recurrent genital ulcers with frequent episodes (4–6 or more per year) or severe, distressing symptoms, suppressive therapy is often preferred over episodic treatment. After a year of suppressive therapy, patients can be reassessed to decide whether they wish to continue or switch to episodic treatment, though they should be informed that recurrence rates may return to pretherapy levels once suppressive treatment stops. For immunocompromised individuals, including those living with HIV, dosage adjustments are necessary for valaciclovir and famciclovir but not for acyclovir. In recurrent cases, valaciclovir is recommended at 500 mg for 5 days instead of 3, while famciclovir should be administered at 500 mg twice daily for

TABLE 1: Treatment of genital herpes and syphilis.

Infection	First-line options	Effective substitutes	For pregnant/breastfeeding women and <16 years
Genital herpes: Primary infection	• Acyclovir 400 mg orally, 3×/day for 10 days • Acyclovir 200 mg orally, 5×/day for 10 days	• Valaciclovir 500 mg twice daily for 10 days • Famciclovir 250 mg orally, 3×/day for 10 days	Use acyclovir only if the benefit outweighs the risk; same dosage as for non-pregnant individuals
Genital herpes: Recurrent infection— episodic	• Acyclovir 400 mg orally, 3×/day for 5 days • Acyclovir 800 mg orally, 2×/day for 5 days • Acyclovir 800 mg orally, 3×/day for 2 days	• Valaciclovir 500 mg twice daily for 5 days • Famciclovir 250 mg orally, 2×/day for 5 days	• Acyclovir 400 mg orally, 3×/day for 5 days • Acyclovir 800 mg orally, 2×/day for 5 days • Acyclovir 800 mg, 3×/day for 2 days
Genital herpes: Suppressive therapy	• Acyclovir 400 mg orally, 2×/day • Valaciclovir 500 mg once daily	Famciclovir 250 mg orally, 2×/day	• Acyclovir 400 mg orally, 2×/day • Valaciclovir 500 mg once daily
Syphilis (early)	Benzathine penicillin 2.4 million units, intramuscularly, single dose	• Doxycycline 100 mg orally, 2×/day for 14 days • Erythromycin 500 mg orally, 4×/day for 14 days	• Benzathine penicillin 2.4 million units, intramuscularly, single dose • Erythromycin 500 mg orally, 4×/day for 14 days
Syphilis (late)	Benzathine penicillin 2.4 million units, intramuscularly, once weekly for 3 weeks	• Procaine penicillin 1.2 million units, intramuscularly, daily for 20 days • Doxycycline 100 mg orally, 2×/day for 30 days	Erythromycin 500 mg orally, 4×/day for 30 days

5 days rather than 250 mg. For suppressive treatment, the recommended dosage for valaciclovir is 500 mg twice daily instead of once, and famciclovir at 500 mg twice daily instead of the standard 250 mg. Additionally, individuals allergic to penicillin should receive alternative treatments for syphilis, such as doxycycline or erythromycin, which are effective substitutes **(Table 1)**.

CONCLUSION

Genital ulcer disease encompasses a diverse group of sexually transmitted infections, each with unique clinical, epidemiological, and diagnostic challenges. Accurate diagnosis is critical, as clinical features alone are often insufficient to distinguish between conditions such as genital herpes, syphilis, chancroid, lymphogranuloma venereum (LGV), and donovanosis. While molecular diagnostic tools like NAAT and PCR offer high sensitivity and specificity, they may not be readily available in all settings, necessitating a syndromic management approach in resource-limited environments.

Early recognition and appropriate treatment of GUD are essential to prevent complications, reduce transmission, and manage co-infections such as HIV.

Suppressive therapy for recurrent herpes, timely intervention in syphilis, and tailored management for LGV and donovanosis are cornerstones of effective care. In endemic areas, public health strategies—including education, routine screening, and improved access to diagnostics—play a crucial role in disease control. Ultimately, a combination of clinical acumen, epidemiological awareness, and evidence-based protocols ensures optimal outcomes for patients with genital ulcer disease.

REFERENCES

1. Kimberlin DW, Rouse DJ. Clinical practice. Genital herpes. N Engl J Med. 2004;350:1970-7.
2. Ayoub HH, Chemaitelly H, Abu-Raddad LJ. Characterizing the transitioning epidemiology of herpes simplex virus type 1 in the USA: Model-based predictions. BMC Med. 2019;17:57.
3. Magdaleno-Tapial J, Hernandez-Bel P, Valenzuela-Onate C, Ortiz-Salvador JM, Garcia-Legaz-Martinez M, Martinez-Domenech A, et al. Genital infection with herpes simplex virus type 1 and type 2 in Valencia, Spain: A retrospective observational study. Actas Dermosifiliogr. 2020;111:53-8.
4. Looker KJ, Welton NJ, Sabin KM, Dalal S, Vickerman P, Turner KME, et al. Global and regional estimates of the contribution of herpes simplex virus type 2 infection to HIV incidence: A population attributable fraction analysis using published epidemiological data. Lancet Infect Dis. 2019;20:240-9.
5. R R, Shome K, Sarkar P, Manna S. Morbidity Profile of Patients With Sexually Transmitted Infections (STIs) and Their Determinants in a Tertiary Care Institute of Eastern India. Cureus. 2025;17(2):e78963.
6. Ghosh A, Panda S, Bhattacharyya S. Seronegative and Low Seropositive Treatment-Naive Secondary Syphilis in India: A Cross Sectional Study. Indian J Dermatol. 2024;69(6):486.
7. Gravett RM, Marrazzo J. An Ulcer by Any Other Name: Non-herpes and Non-syphilis Ulcerative Sexually Transmitted Infections. Infect Dis Clin North Am. 2023;37(2):369-80.
8. Cunha Ramos M, Nicola MRC, Bezerra NTC, Sardinha JCG, Sampaio de Souza Morais J, Schettini AP. Genital ulcers caused by sexually transmitted agents. An Bras Dermatol. 2022;97(5):551-65.
9. Szumowski JD, Marquez C. Lymphogranuloma venereum as a cause of persistent perianal ulcers. BMJ Case Rep. 2021;14(2):e240551.
10. Belda Junior W. Donovanosis. An Bras Dermatol. 2020;95(6):675-683.

CHAPTER 3

Discharge

Sudip Das, Apeksha Singh

INTRODUCTION

Normal Vaginal Discharge

Normal vaginal discharge is typically whitish, nonmalodorous, and floccular in consistency. Its amount varies among individuals, with a normal pH ranging from 3.5 to 4.5, maintained by Döderlein's lactobacilli.[1] These bacilli convert glycogen into lactic acid, creating an acidic environment. The cellular components include sloughed cells from the cervical columnar and vaginal squamous epithelium, serous vaginal transudate, and cervical mucus, along with water, electrolytes, facultative microorganisms, fatty acids, proteins, and carbohydrates.[1]

Features indicating abnormal discharge:[1]
- Hypervaginal secretion unrelated to menstruation
- Offensive or malodorous discharge
- Yellowish discharge

Normal vaginal flora healthy vaginal flora consists of:
- *Lactobacillus* species
- Anaerobic gram-negative bacilli
- Bacteroides, streptococci, *Candida albicans*, and others

Abnormal Vaginal Discharge

Abnormal vaginal discharge may result from physiological or pathological causes.

Physiological causes:
- Age-dependent variations (neonates, prepuberty, and childbearing)
- Conditions such as pregnancy and sexual arousal

Pathological causes:
- Noninfective factors, such as foreign bodies [e.g., tampons and intrauterine contraceptive device (IUCD)], chemical irritants, and gynecological conditions (e.g., endocervical polyps and tumors) **(Fig. 1)**.
- Infective conditions, including bacterial vaginosis (BV), candidiasis, and trichomoniasis **(Flowchart 1)**.

Bacterial Vaginosis

Bacterial vaginosis is the most common cause of vaginal discharge among women attending gynecological clinics **(Figs. 2A and B)**. It involves a loss of the normal vaginal ecosystem and a shift to a mixed flora dominated by anaerobic bacteria, including *Gardnerella vaginalis, Mobiluncus,* and *Prevotella* species.[2]

Clinical Features

- Malodorous discharge
- Elevated vaginal pH (>4.5)
- Thin, homogenous discharge
- Positive amine test ("whiff test")

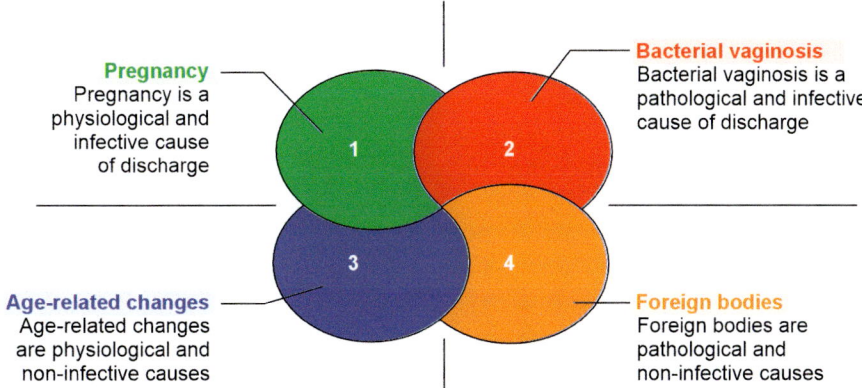

FIG. 1: Causes of abnormal vaginal discharge classified by physiological/pathological and infective/noninfective nature.

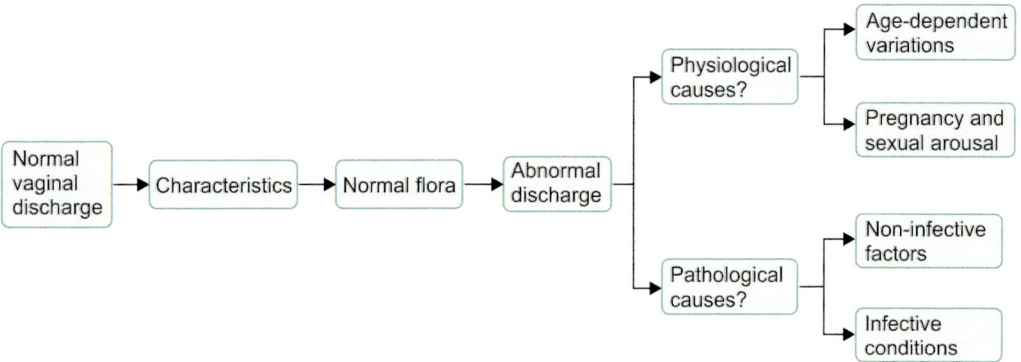

FLOWCHART 1: Flowchart showing progression from normal to abnormal vaginal discharge based on characteristics, flora, and physiological or pathological causes.

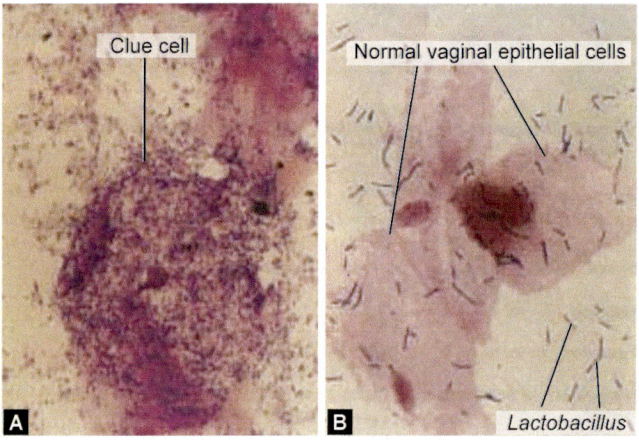

FIGS. 2A AND B: Clue cells indicating bacterial vaginosis.

Diagnosis
- Amsel's clinical criteria
- Nugent scoring (Gram staining)

Amsel's clinical criteria: Diagnosis requires three or more of the following clinical/diagnostic features:
- Excessive homogeneous uniformly adherent vaginal discharge
- Elevated vaginal pH > 4.5
- Positive amine test (Whiff test)
- Clue cells (20%)

Bacterial Vaginosis and Pregnancy
- Associated with adverse outcomes like preterm birth
- Treated with metronidazole or clindamycin
- BV during pregnancy is associated with adverse pregnancy outcomes, including PROM, preterm labor, preterm birth, postpartum endometritis, and intra-amniotic infections.

Human Immunodeficiency Virus and Bacterial Vaginosis
Bacterial vaginosis might enhance the susceptibility to HIV infection.

Treatment
All symptomatic pregnant women should be tested and treated:
- Metronidazole 250 mg orally three times a day for 7 days, or
- Metronidazole 500 mg orally twice a day for 7 days, or
- Clindamycin 300 mg orally twice a day for 7 days
- Metronidazole is not recommended for use in the first trimester of pregnancy, but it may be used during the second and third trimesters.
- Currently, pregnant women with asymptomatic bacterial vaginosis are not routinely screened or treated.
- Partner treatment not recommended

- Culture is the "gold standard" for diagnosis of trichomoniasis.
- It is especially of use when the organism load is low, e.g., in asymptomatic women.

Various media have been used to detect trichomonas, such as:
- Diamond (trypticase, yeast, and maltose)
- Modified diamond
- Lash, NIH, and Feinberg–Whittington media
- Cultures are seldom used for diagnosis in routine situations.

Management of Sex Partners
- Sex partners of patients with *Trichomonas vaginalis* should be treated.
- Patients should be instructed to avoid sex until they and their sex partners are cured.

Trichomoniasis
Trichomoniasis is caused by the protozoan *Trichomonas vaginalis*. It is primarily sexually transmitted, with high transmission rates from men to women **(Table 1)**.

Clinical Features
- Copious, malodorous yellow–green discharge
- Elevated vaginal pH
- Strawberry cervix (colpitis macularis)

Diagnosis and Treatment
- Diagnosed using direct microscopy, culture, or fluorescent antibody techniques
- Treat patients and their partners to prevent reinfection

Trichomoniasis Association with Human Immunodeficiency Virus
The associations between HIV and trichomoniasis, similar to other sexually transmitted diseases (STDs), may relate to:
- Increased shedding of HIV because of the local inflammation produced by the STDs

- Increased susceptibility to HIV because of the macroscopic or microscopic breaks in mucosal barriers caused by the STDs

Reproductive complications in women include:
- Risk factor for transmission of HIV
- Associated with pelvic inflammatory disease (PID)
- Greater risk for tubal infertility
- Associated with preterm birth and low birth weight
- Increased risk of post-hysterectomy infection
- Risk factor for cervical neoplasia

Management of Sex Partners
- Sex partners of patients with *T. vaginalis* should be treated.
- Patients should be instructed to avoid sex until they and their sex partners are cured.

Vulvovaginal Candidiasis

Caused mostly by *Candida albicans*, vulvovaginal candidiasis (VVC) is characterized by pruritus, soreness, and curdy white discharge **(Fig. 3)**. It can be uncomplicated or complicated, depending on frequency, severity, and the patient's immune status.[4,5]

Clinical Features
- Thick, cottage cheese-like discharge
- Minimal odor
- Vaginal and vulvar irritation

Diagnosis
- Microscopic examination (KOH preparation)
- Vaginal culture

Treatment
- Short-course topical azoles for uncomplicated cases
- Extended therapy for recurrent VVC

TABLE 1: CDC recommendation for trichomoniasis.[3]

Risk category	Recommended regimen	Alternatives
Women	Metronidazole 500 mg twice daily for 7 days	Tinidazole 2 g orally in a single dose
Men	Metronidazole 2 g orally in a single dose	Tinidazole 2 g orally in a single dose

(CDC: Centers for Disease Control and Prevention)

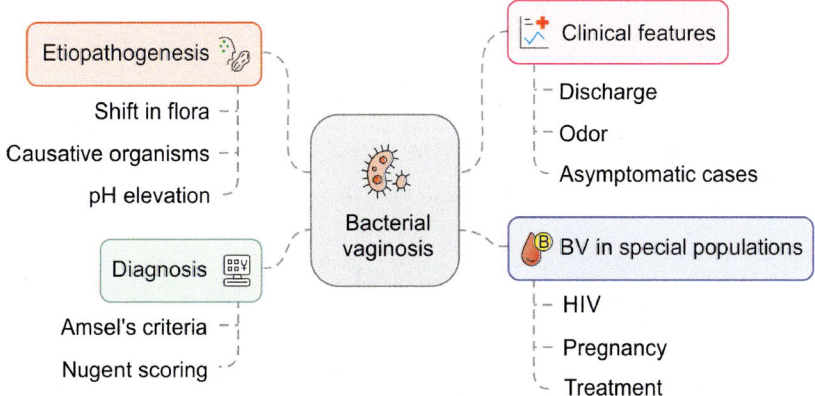

FIG. 3: Overview of bacterial vaginosis: Etiopathogenesis, diagnosis, clinical features, and management in special populations.

Cervicitis

Cervicitis can be classified into:
- *Endocervicitis*: Often caused by *Chlamydia trachomatis* or *Neisseria gonorrhoeae*
- *Ectocervicitis*: Associated with *HSV* and *Trichomonas vaginalis*

Clinical Features
- Purulent endocervical discharge
- Abnormal menstrual bleeding

Diagnosis
Swab tests, Gram staining, and nucleic acid amplification test (NAAT) for pathogens.

Management
Treat sexual partners to prevent reinfection **(Fig. 4)**.

Follow-up: Monitor treatment response and address recurrent symptoms

URETHRAL DISCHARGE

Definition
Urethritis refers to inflammation of the urethra, typically presenting with urethral discharge, dysuria (painful urination), or pruritus at the urethral meatus. It can be caused by infectious or noninfectious etiologies, with sexually transmitted infections (STIs) being the most common cause in young adults **(Fig. 5)**.

Classification
Urethritis can be broadly classified into:[4,5]
- *Gonococcal urethritis (GU)*—caused by *Neisseria gonorrhoeae*
- *Nongonococcal urethritis (NGU)*—caused by other pathogens, most commonly *Chlamydia trachomatis* (20-50%), *Ureaplasma urealyticum* (10-20%), *Mycoplasma genitalium* (10-20%), *Trichomonas vaginalis* (1-17%), herpes simplex virus (HSV), *Adenovirus Candida* species, *Coliform bacteria*, *Staphylococcus saprophyticus*, *Haemophilus* species, *Neisseria meningitidis*, and *Streptococcus pneumoniae*
- *Noninfective causes*: Urethral stricture, catheterization, congenital abnormalities of the urogenital system, Stevens–Johnson syndrome, chemical irritation (from douches, lubricants, etc.), tumors,

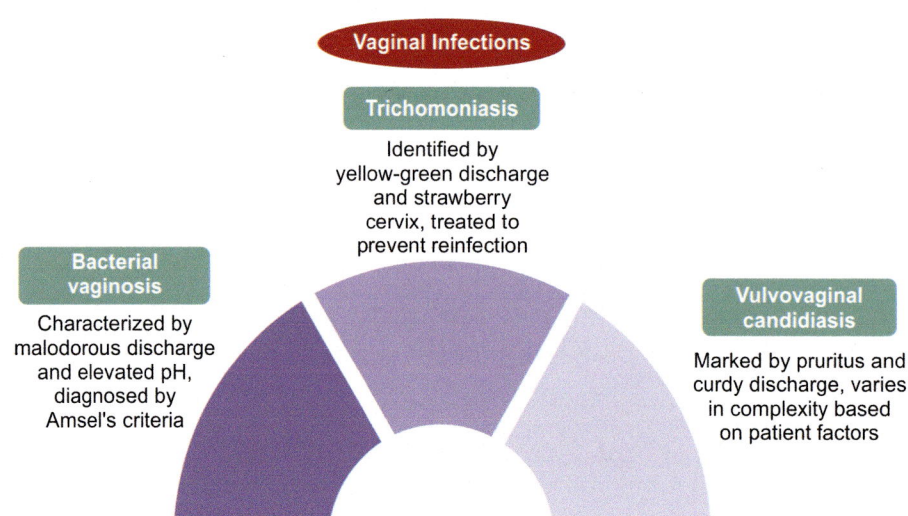

FIG. 4: Different causes of vaginal discharge infective causes.

foreign bodies (especially in children and teenagers), and condom allergy **(Fig. 6)**.

Gonococcal Urethritis

Etiology
- Caused by *Neisseria gonorrhoeae*, a gram-negative, intracellular, oxidase-positive diplococcus[2]
- Ferments glucose but not maltose

Pathogenesis
- Organism attaches to and invades mucosal surfaces (columnar and transitional epithelium)

- Infection typically involves the urethra, cervix, rectum, pharynx, and conjunctiva.[6]
- *Mechanism involves*:
    - *Adherence* via pili and Opa proteins
    - *Invasion* into epithelial cells
    - *Tissue damage* due to immune response and bacterial enzymes

Clinical Features
In males:
- Purulent, thick, yellow or white urethral discharge **(Fig. 7)**
- Dysuria, increased frequency of urination
- Occasionally penile edema ("bull-head clap")
- May be asymptomatic in ~10%

In females:
- Cervicitis is the most common presentation.
- Dysuria, urgency, and scanty mucopurulent discharge
- Erythema and edema at the cervical ectopy
- Postcoital or induced bleeding

Rectal gonorrhea:
- Seen in receptive anal intercourse or secondary to genital infection
- *Symptoms*: Anal pruritus, discharge, proctitis, tenesmus, and constipation

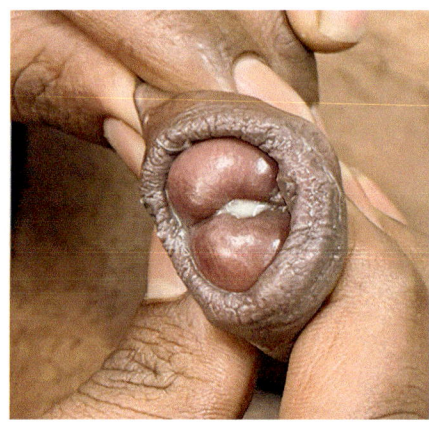

FIG. 5: Clinical picture of urethral discharge.

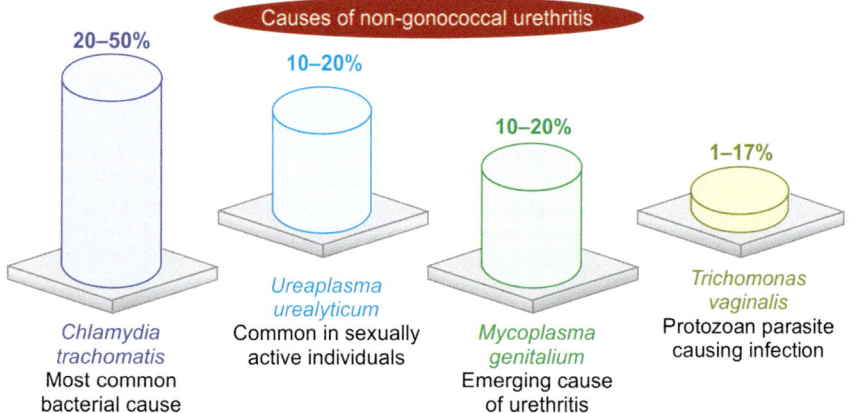

FIG. 6: Different causes of nongonococcal urethritis infective causes.

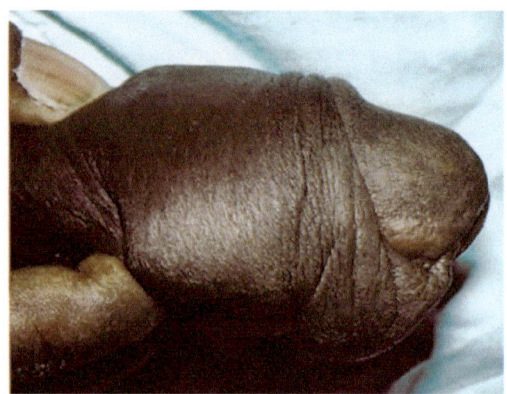

FIG. 7: Swelling of distal shaft showing bull head clap.

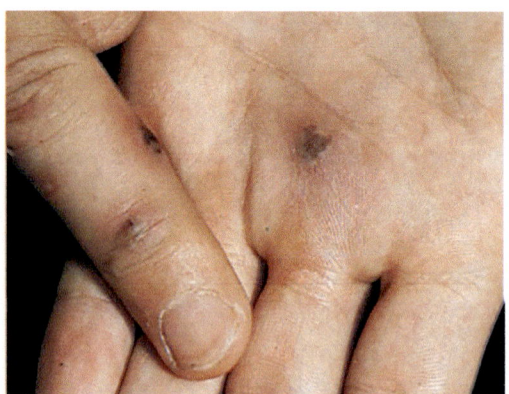

FIG. 8: Disseminated gonococcal infection—tender, hemorrhagic pustules on the fingers and palms.

Pharyngeal gonorrhea:
- May cause acute pharyngitis, tonsillitis, cervical lymphadenopathy
- Often asymptomatic

Complications

In males:
- Posterior urethritis
- Epididymitis
- Prostatitis
- Seminal vesiculitis
- Periurethral abscess (→ "watering-can perineum")

In females:
- Pelvic inflammatory disease
- Salpingitis → infertility
- Bartholin's gland abscess

In infants: Ophthalmia neonatorum (gonococcal conjunctivitis acquired during childbirth)

Metastatic complications: Disseminated gonococcal infection (DGI)—
- Migratory polyarthritis
- Tenosynovitis
- Dermatitis (macules, pustules, petechiae, and bullae)
- *Rarely*: Endocarditis, meningitis, and perihepatitis **(Fig. 8)**

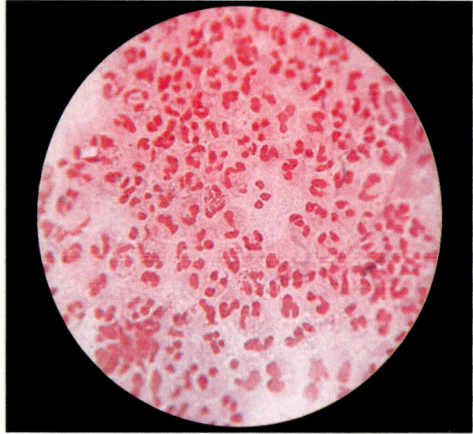

FIG. 9: Microscopy showing ICDC (intracellular diplococci).

Diagnosis

- *Microscopy*: Gram stain—intracellular gram-negative diplococci in polymorphonuclear leukocytes (PMNs) **(Fig. 9)**
- *Culture*:
   - Thayer–Martin, NYC medium
   - *Colonies*: Round, translucent, and convex
- *Nucleic acid amplification tests (NAATs)*: Preferred for sensitivity/specificity
- *Serology*: Enzyme-linked immunosorbent assay (ELISA) and radioimmunoassay (RIA) (rarely used)

Treatment of Gonococcal Urethritis

Centers for Disease Control and Prevention (CDC)/National AIDS Control Organization (NACO) guidelines:[3] Ceftriaxone 500 mg IM single dose + Doxycycline 100 mg BID × 7 days if *Chlamydia* not excluded

Nongonococcal Urethritis

Common Causes
- *Chlamydia trachomatis* (most common)
- *Ureaplasma urealyticum*
- *Mycoplasma genitalium*
- *Trichomonas vaginalis*
- Herpes simplex virus (HSV)
- Adenovirus

Chlamydial Urethritis

Pathogen characteristics: Obligate intracellular, gram-negative bacterium **(Fig. 10)**
- *Exists in two forms:*
  - *Elementary body*: Infectious form
  - *Reticulate body*: Replicative form

Clinical Features

In men:
- Dysuria, mild whitish or mucoid discharge

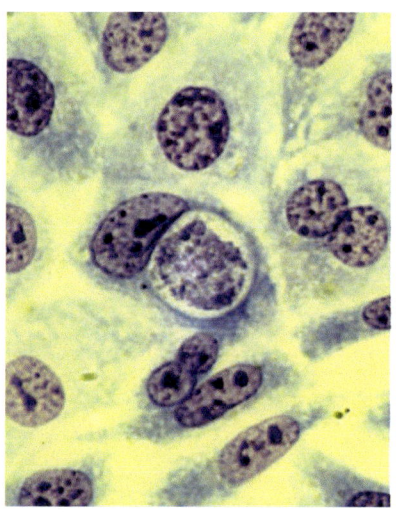

FIG. 10: Cell infected with *Chlamydia* showing perinuclear draped inclusion body.

- Focal tenderness of urethra
- May mimic herpetic lesions
- *Complications*: Epididymitis, prostatitis, and proctitis **(Figs. 11A and B)**

In women:
- *Cervicitis*: Mucopurulent discharge, ectopy, and cervical bleeding
- PID, salpingitis
- *Urethritis*: Dysuria and frequency
- *Pregnancy*: Risk of abortion, low birth weight (LBW), neonatal conjunctivitis/pneumonia

Diagnosis of Chlamydial Urethritis
- *Gram stain*: ≥2 PMNs/OIF
- *Giemsa stain*: Basophilic intracytoplasmic inclusions
- *Iodine stain*: Brown bodies
- *NAATs*: Preferred
- *Cell culture*: McCoy or HeLa cells (less common)

Treatment

CDC guidelines:[3] Doxycycline 100 mg BID × 7 days or Azithromycin 1 g single dose.

Other Infectious Causes

Ureaplasma urealyticum:
- Linked to urethritis, prostatitis, and PID
- Cultured in pleuropneumonia-like organism (PPLO) broth
- Treated with doxycycline or azithromycin

Mycoplasma genitalium:
- Common in recurrent NGU
- *Diagnosis*: NAATs
- *Treatment*: Azithromycin or moxifloxacin (if resistant)

Trichomonas vaginalis:
- Flagellated protozoa, often co-infects with NG or CT **(Fig. 12)**
- *Diagnosis*: Wet mount and NAATs
- *Treatment*: Metronidazole or tinidazole 2 g orally, single dose

Persistent and recurrent NGU:
- *Persistent*: ≥29 days post-treatment

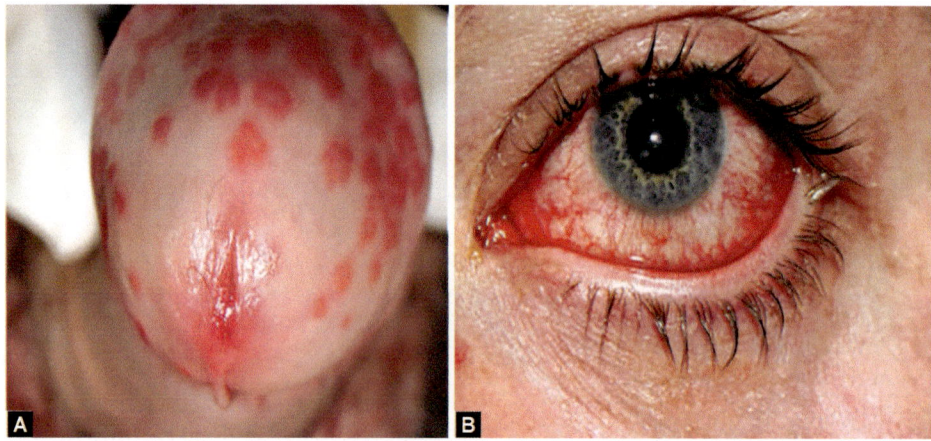

FIGS. 11A AND B: (A) Penile discharge and (B) conjunctivitis caused by *Chlamydia trachomatis*.

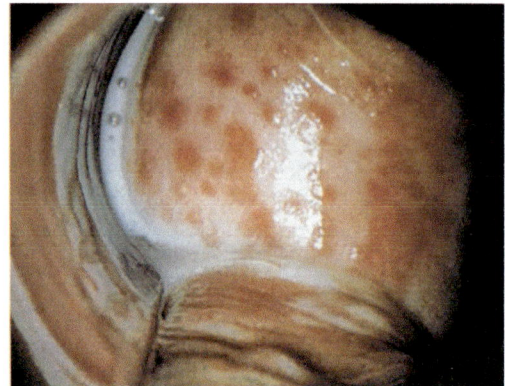

FIG. 12: Strawberry appearance of cervix caused by trichomonas vaginalis.

- *Recurrent*: Recurrence between 30 and 92 days
- *Causes*: Reinfection, drug resistance, *M. genitalium*, and *T. vaginalis*

- *Management*:
    - Repeat NAATs
    - Consider alternate regimens
    - Ensure partner notification and treatment

CONCLUSION

Discharge is a common STI manifestation and must be approached with thorough clinical evaluation and sensitive diagnostic tools. Empirical treatment following national or international guidelines, partner management, and patient education is key to preventing recurrence and complications **(Table 2)**.

TABLE 2: Syndromic approach (KITS) to urethral and vaginal/cervical discharge.

Urethral discharge	Cervical discharge	Painful scrotal swelling	Vaginal discharge
• Urethral discharge (pus or mucopurulent) • Pain or burning while passing urine • Increased frequency of urination • Systemic symptoms such as malaise and fever	• Nature and type of discharge (quantity, color, and odor) • Burning while passing urine, increased frequency • Genital complaints by sexual partners • Low backache (Take menstrual history to rule out pregnancy)	• Swelling and pain in scrotal region • Pain or burning while passing urine • Systemic symptoms such as malaise and fever • History of urethral discharge	• Nature and type of discharge (quantity, color, and odor) • Burning while passing urine and increased frequency • Genital complaints by sexual partners • Low backache (Take menstrual history to rule out pregnancy)
Tablet Azithromycin 1 g OD stat + Tablet Cefixime 400 mg OD stat	Tablet Azithromycin 1 g OD stat + Tablet Cefixime 400 mg OD stat	Tablet Azithromycin 1 g OD stat + Tablet Cefixime 400 mg OD stat	Tablet Secnidazole 2 g OD stat + Capsule Fluconazole 150 mg OD Stat
KIT 1/Gray	KIT 1/Gray	KIT 1/Gray	KIT 2/Green
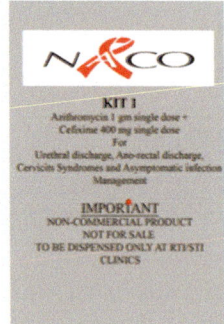	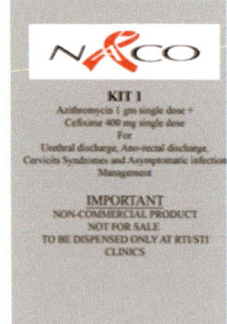	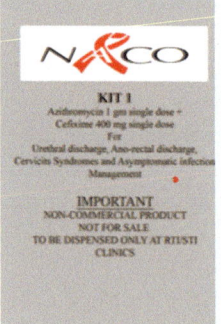	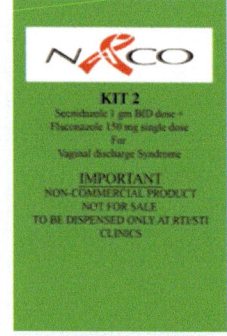
Treat all recent partners	Treat partners when symptomatic	Treat all recent partners	Treat partners when symptomatic

REFERENCES

1. Willcox RR, Willcox JR. Venereological medicine. In: Gupta S, Kumar B (Eds). Sexually Transmitted Infections, 2nd edition. Amsterdam: Elsevier: 2012.
2. Sharma VK. Textbook of Sexually Transmitted Diseases and HIV/AIDS, 2nd edition. New Delhi: Viva Books; 2012.
3. Centers for Disease Control and Prevention. Sexually transmitted infections treatment guidelines, 2021. MMWR Recomm Rep. 2021;70(4):1-187.
4. Thappa DM, Kumari R. Establishment of IADVL and its present day status. Indian J Dermatol Venereol Leprol. 2009;75:204.
5. Bodey GP. Candidiasis: Pathogenesis, Diagnosis and Treatment, 2nd edition. Philadelphia: Lippincott Williams and Wilkins; 1992.
6. Holmes KK. Sexually transmitted diseases, 4th edition. New York: Mc Graw Hill Education; 2008.

CHAPTER 4

Anogenital Warts

Konakanchi Venkata Chalam, Padmasri Somala Y

INTRODUCTION

Anogenital warts, condyloma acuminata, or genital warts are the benign proliferation of anogenital mucosa caused by infection with human papillomavirus (HPV). There are about 200 types of HPV of which >40 can infect the anogenital region and is mainly transmitted by sexual contact but rarely can also be transmitted by nonsexual contact.

Clinically, it manifests as warty skin-colored or flesh-colored papules or plaques in the vulva, vagina, and cervix regions of females, penile and scrotal regions of males, and pubic, groin, and perianal areas of both males and females.[1]

Anogenital warts were considered a manifestation of syphilis in the 15th century but in 1980 Gissman and Zur Hausen, isolated HPV type 6. Zur Hausen also isolated HPV16 and HPV18 in cervical cancers in 1983–1984 for which he received the Noble Prize in 2008.[2]

EPIDEMIOLOGY

- HPV as an etiological agent is the most common sexually transmitted infection (STI) in the world. In the United States, at least 75% of sexually active individuals have been infected with at least one type of HPV. The prevalence rate in the USA is 10–20% in unvaccinated individuals and prevalence decreases if vaccination is implemented.[3]
- In India, the current prevalence of genital warts is approximately 1.07%. The prevalence is higher in males (1.22%) versus females (0.99%). The highest prevalence has been noticed in Delhi (2.17%) followed by Hyderabad (1.35%) and Kolkata (1.21%).[4]
- The incubation period varies from 3 months to 24 months. The incidence of infection is high in 16–24 years of age group and common in males compared to females.[5]
- Anogenital warts are not common in children but children presenting with anogenital warts should be evaluated for sexual abuse.

ETIOPATHOGENESIS

Flowchart 1 shows pathogenesis of anogenital warts.
- Anogenital warts are caused by the HPV. HPV is a nonenveloped double-stranded DNA virus belonging to the family Papovaviridae which infects the stratified squamous epithelium of the skin and mucous membrane.
- Human papillomavirus is a small nonenveloped capsid virus with an 8 kilobase genome composed of six early open reading frames (E1, E2, E4, E5, E6, and E7) and late open reading frames L1 and L2.

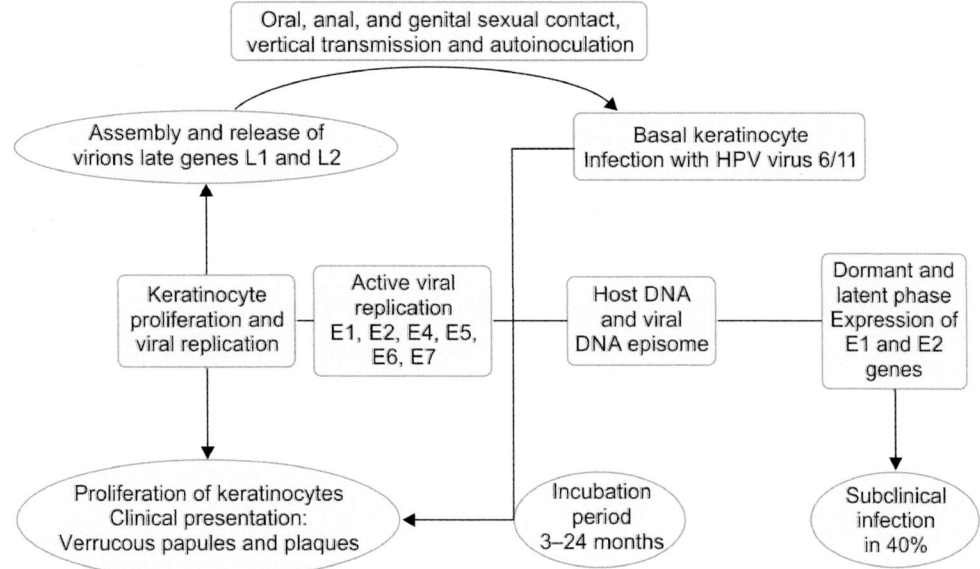

FLOWCHART 1: Pathogenesis of genital warts.

- The early-open E genes are important for regulatory function and encode proteins involved in viral replication and cell transformation. The late-open L genes encode viral capsid proteins L1 and L2 genes code for encapsulating proteins L1 and L2.[3]
- L1 capsid protein is predominantly expressed in artificial cell culture systems, and it self-assembles in the absence of viral genome to form virus-like particles (VLP).[5] This VLP of L1 capsid protein is used in HPV vaccines to induce immunity. L2 is the minor capsid protein and along with L1, it mediates infectivity.[6,7]
- Genital HPV types are divided into high-risk and low-risk groups of viruses depending on the nature of lesions, whether benign or malignant lesion. In low-risk HPV subtypes, they remain separate from host cell DNA and undergo independent replication whereas in high-risk subtypes the viral DNA integrates with host cell DNA and inactivates tumor suppressor genes like *p53* and *Rb* gene leading to risk of malignant transformation.[8]
- HPV 6 and 11 types of viruses are commonly detected in 90% of cases of anogenital warts. The International Agency for Research on Cancer (IARC) has classified HPV subtypes 16/18/31/33/35/39/45/51/52/56/58/59 under the high-risk category.[9-11] Coinfection with high and low-risk types of viruses is also common.
- Anogenital warts caused by HPV types 6 and 11 will remain benign. Apart from genital warts, HPV types 6 and 11 also cause laryngeal papilloma and verrucous carcinoma (CA). Children who acquire infection through nonsexual contact, HPV types 2, 27, and 57 are identified.

TRANSMISSION[12-14]

- Anogenital HPV is predominantly transmitted through sexual, anal, and genital contact in adults. In children, the HPV virus can be rarely transmitted

by nonsexual contact through autoinoculation.
- The risk of infection is approximately 75% after unprotected sexual contact with an infected person. This high rate of transmission generates a 50% lifetime risk of acquiring anogenital warts in sexually active individuals.
- Due to high viral load, subclinical infection can also transmit the infection to uninfected persons.
- Risk factors for the acquisition of infection are early age of sexual activity, multiple sexual partners, unprotected sexual intercourse, use of oral contraceptive pills, history of other STIs, and immunosuppression.
- In immunosuppressed individuals, there is the development of larger lesions, lesions are resistant to treatment, have high recurrence rates, and are likely to transform malignant due to coinfection with high-risk types.
- Smoking increases the risk of acquiring of virus, circumcision decreases the risk of acquiring the virus.
- Transmission in children can be hetero inoculation due to nonsexual contact by caregivers, autoinoculation from the cutaneous infection, sexual abuse, perinatal transmission during vaginal delivery through infected maternal genital tract or fomites such as contaminated towels, underwear, etc.

CLINICAL MANIFESTATIONS[10,11]

- After infection, the incubation period varies from 3 weeks to 8 months. The average duration for the appearance of warts after the initial infection is approximately 2–3 months.
- In 40% of cases, the virus can remain dormant in the infected epithelia without clinical manifestations. Approximately, 30% of cases will undergo spontaneous resolution within the first four months of infection.
- The remission rate is highly variable, and the majority of cases are recurrent even after appropriate treatment. Conversely, the presence of CD4+ lymphocytes in the epidermis and dermis has been associated with an elevated rate of spontaneous regression.
- Anogenital warts are typically found on the anal and genital area including the groin, perineum, vulva, labia, penis, scrotum, perianal region, and suprapubic skin. Internally, they may present in the urethra or cervix or vagina or anal canal up to and below the dentate line.
- Lesions can present as discrete small papules or solitary large masses in the genital and anal areas. Lesions appear as single or multiple flat or dome-shaped, filiform, fungating, pedunculated, verrucous, or cauliflower-like growths. Color varies from white, skin-colored, brown, erythematous, violaceous, or hyperpigmented lesions **(Fig. 1)**.
- The size of lesions varies from a few millimeters to several centimeters in diameter. Extensive condyloma acuminatae can cause disfigurement

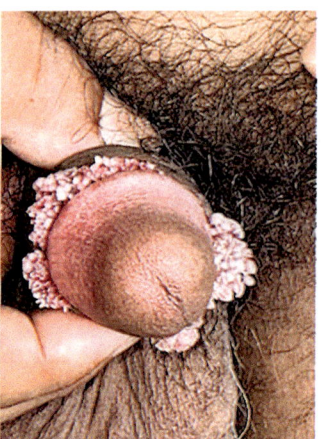

FIG. 1: Genital warts in male—picture depicting cauliflower-like verrucous growth over the prepuce.

of genitalia and may interfere with defecation. Urethral warts may cause urinary obstruction, dysuria, and urethral bleeding.
- When lesions spread and cover the entire anogenital area, it is called a Buschke–Lowenstein tumor which is a premalignant condition arising from condyloma accuminata.
- Lesions are usually asymptomatic but sometimes may cause itching, redness, or discomfort and larger lesions may be subject to bleeding after irritation or contact during intercourse or mechanical irritation. They may also lead to mechanical obstruction which hinders normal vaginal delivery.
- Genital warts can lead to psychological distress and patients may often experience stigmatization, anxiety, depression guilt, and concern about future fertility and cancer risk. Emotional impact on sexual partners can lead to conflict and relationship termination. Proper counseling should be done for these patients.[15]

HISTOPATHOLOGY[10,11]

- Histopathologically, the hallmark of an HPV-infected cell is the development of morphologically atypical keratinocytes known as koilocytes. These are enlarged cells with eccentric, pyknotic nuclei that are often surrounded by a perinuclear halo.
- The epidermis will show a marked acanthosis with varying degrees of papillomatosis, hyperkeratosis, and parakeratosis as well as a complete effacement of the granular cell layer.
- Rete ridges tend to be elongated and point inward toward the center of the wart.
- Dermis will often display an increased vascularization with the presence of thrombosed capillaries.

DERMOSCOPY

Dermoscopy of anogenital warts mainly depicts two features morphological pattern and vascular pattern with papillomatosis.[16]
1. *Morphological pattern*: Knob-like or finger-like pattern
2. *Vascular pattern*: Dotted or glomerular

EVALUATION

Condylomata is commonly diagnosed clinically, but a definitive diagnosis is made by polymerase chain reaction (PCR).

TREATMENT[10,11]

- There are different modalities for treating anogenital warts and usually, the treatment modalities are focused on removing the wart tissue rather than eradicating the underlying infection.
- According to present data, there is no definitive therapy labeled as the best standard of care for CA.
- The therapy of choice depends on the cost, side effect profile, efficacy and duration of treatment, and the patient's choice.
- CA is treated in the following ways:[17]
  - *Application of topical agents*: Podophyllotoxin, imiquimod, sinecatechins, podophyllin, and 5 fluorouracil **(Table 1)**
  - *Intralesional*: Bleomycin injection, interferons (IFN-α), immunotherapy [bacillus Calmette–Guérin, measles, mumps, and rubella, and purified protein derivative (BCG, MMR, PPD), and *Candida* antigen] **(Table 2)**
  - *Surgical and destructive methods*: Cryotherapy, electrosurgery, scissor excision, CO_2 laser, and trichloroacetic acid
  - *Systemic treatment*: IFNs, isotretinoin, and low-dose cyclophosphamide

TABLE 1: Patient applied treatment modalities for treatment of genital warts.[11]

Treatment modality	Podophyllotoxin (0.5% solution or gel and 0.15% cream)	Imiquimod 5% cream	Sinecatechins 15% ointment	5 fluorouracil 5% cream
Mechanism of action	Binds to the cellular microtubules and inhibits mitotic division	Activate the immune cells leads to the secretion of multiple cytokines such as interferons-α, interleukin 6, and tumor necrosis factor-α	• Modulate the inflammatory response through inhibition of transcription factors AP-1 and NF-kB. • Antitumor, antiviral, and antioxidant	Inhibits key enzymes in DNA replication
Administered by	Patient	Patient	Patient	Patient
Dosing schedule	Twice daily for 3 consecutive days of the week (maximum 4 weeks)	Applied at bedtime three times per week for up to 16 weeks	Applied to warts three times a day for up to 4 months	• One to two times/day till resolution of lesions • Used for urethral warts
Precautions	• Area of application < 10 cm² • Total volume applied/day < 0.5 mL • Washed off after 1–4 hours	Should be on the skin for 6–10 hours and later washed with soap and water	If the patient is not responding within a few weeks the modality should be changed	–
Pregnancy/Lactation	Contraindicated	Contraindicated	Contraindicated	Contraindicated
Adverse effects	Pain, inflammation, erosion, burning, and itching	• *Common*: Itching, erythema, burning, ulceration, irritation, and pain • *Systemic*: Headache, myalgia, fatigue, and malaise	• *Common*: Redness, burning, itching, and pain • *Rare*: Lymphadenitis, vulvovaginitis, balanitis, and ulceration	Teratogenicity, local soreness, erythema, and ulceration
Clearance rate	45–77%	56%	58%	10–50%
Recurrence rate	38–65%	13%	6–9%	50%

(AP: activator protein-1; NF-kB: nuclear factor-kappa B)

TABLE 2: Physician applied topical and intralesional modalities for treatment of genital warts.[11]

Treatment modality	Podophyllin 25% tincture of benzoin	Trichloroacetic acid solution (80–100%)	Bleomycin injection	Interferons (IFN-α)	Immunotherapy (BCG, MMR, PPD, Candida antigen)
Mechanism of action	Binds to the cellular microtubules and inhibits mitotic division	Chemical cautery	Antimitotic agent	Antiviral	Increases immunity against the virus
Administered by	Physician	Physician	Physician	Physician	Physician
Dosing schedule	Applied twice weekly	Weekly once	<2 mL/session, 1 mg/mL concentration given intralesional	1–1.5 million units. Intralesional three times weekly for 3 weeks	Once in 3–4 weeks intralesional
Precautions	• Podophyllin is no longer recommended due to high levels of mutagens • Should not be applied to areas > 110 mm² • Side effects are minimized by applying a thin layer and solution is allowed to air dry completely	Not applied for intrameatal warts	• The maximum dose should not exceed 2 mL per session • Should not be given in peripheral vascular disease	Should not be given in bone marrow suppression, psychiatric illness, and major systemic dysfunction	HIV patients, immunosuppression, hypersensitivity to antigen
Pregnancy/Lactation	Contraindicated	Safe in pregnancy	Contraindicated	Category C	Contraindicated
Adverse effects	Local effects are the same as podophyllotoxin. Systemic side effects include fever, mild gastrointestinal distress, paralytic ileus, bone marrow suppression, polyneuritis, paresthesia, coma, and death	Local ulceration Meatal stenosis	Depigmentation, pain, and crusting.	Flu-like symptoms, depression, and pancytopenia	Localized burning, ulceration, and flu-like symptoms
Clearance rate	42–50%	64–88%	14–95%	44.4%	0–88
Recurrence rate	46–60%	19–29%	Not available	21%	Not available

(BCG: bacillus Calmette–Guérin; MMR: measles, mumps, and rubella; PPD: purified protein derivative)

Cryotherapy

- *Mechanism of action:* Infected tissue is frozen with the use of a cooling agent liquid nitrogen, resulting in the initiation of immune response and clearance of warts. Cryotherapy is effective for small and multiple lesions on the vulva and penis.
- Done by a physician, 2–3 freeze-thaw cycles per visit
- *Side effects*: Pain, blistering, ulceration, permanent scarring of tissue, and skin depigmentation
- *Pregnancy and lactation*: Safe
- *Clearance rate*: 79–88%
- *Recurrence rate*: 25–40%

Electrosurgery–Electrofulguration

- *Mechanism of action:* High-frequency electric current causes thermal coagulation and electrocautery will burn and destroy the lesion. Useful to treat small lesions on the shaft of the penis, and vulva and is not recommended for large lesions due to scarring. Done by a physician under local anesthesia.
- *Side effects*: Pain, scarring of tissue, and skin depigmentation
- Contraindicated in patients with cardiac pacemakers
- *Pregnancy and lactation*: Safe
- *Clearance rate*: 94%

Surgical Scissor Excision

It is the oldest modality of treatment. This involves the removal of warty tissue with a scissor or blade and suturing the healthy skin. It is a painful procedure and it should be done under local anesthesia.

- *Clearance rate:* 72%
- It is not the treatment modality of choice nowadays, but it is used in treating large warts which do not respond to conventional methods and in treating intrameatal warts.
- It is useful in the removal of large warts with suspicion of neoplasm to follow-up histopathologically.
- *Limitations:* Painful process requires local or general anesthesia, bleeding, and scarring.

CO_2 Laser Therapy

- *Mechanism of action:* Concentrated beam of laser light energy destroys the target tissue. Light coagulates the vessels which provide a complete bloodless field. Laser permits precise tissue ablation resulting in rapid healing with little scar formation.
- Side effects are minimal, limited to the burning of normal tissue surrounding the lesion
- Good treatment option in immunosuppressed individuals and pregnant women.
- *Demerits:* Laser therapy is very expensive and requires additional training to utilize equipment effectively. Laser vaporization of viral lesions releases viral particles into the surrounding environment. Careful precautions should be taken by physicians and assisting persons to protect from infection of the respiratory tract. Genital warts carry high-risk HPV types which impose a greater risk of transmission of high-risk types.

Systemic Treatment

- IFN-α has been used predominantly for the treatment of malignant melanoma; IFN therapy can be administered systemically, via oral or intramuscular injection, as well as locally, via direct intralesional injections. The use of IFN therapy for the treatment of genital warts remains controversial.
- *Mechanism of action*: Direct immune-boosting effects will promote the clearance of underlying virally infected cells
- *Side effects*: Flu-like symptoms, such as headache, nausea, vomiting, fatigue,

TABLE 3: Human papillomavirus (HPV) vaccines.[10,11]

	CERVARIX Bivalent HPV recombinant vaccine	GARDASIL Quadri-valent HPV recombinant vaccine	GARDASIL 9 9-valent HPV recombinant vaccine
Type of HPV for which the vaccine provides protection	16, 18-cervical cancer, CIN grade 1 or worse, cervical adenocarcinoma in situ	• 6, 11—genital warts • 16, 18-cervical, vulvar, vaginal cancers, CIN grade 1 or worse, and cervical adenocarcinoma	• 6,11—genital warts • 16, 18, 31, 33, 45, 52, and 58-cervical, vulvar, vaginal cancers, CIN grade 1 or worse, and cervical adenocarcinoma
Gender/Age	Females 9–26 years	Males and females 9–26 years	Males and females 9–26 years
Dosing schedule	Three dose series 0, 1, and 6 months	Three dose series 0, 2, and 6 months	Three dose series 0, 2, and 6 months

myalgia, elevated liver enzymes, bone marrow suppression, bronchospasms, and depression

PREVENTION[10,11]

- *Condoms*: Do not offer 100% protection.
- Sexual abstinence
- Limiting the number of sexual partners
- *Vaccination:* HPV vaccine protects from HPV infection and further development of benign and malignant tumors. Cervarix, Gardasil, and Gardasil 9 are the safe types of vaccines available for prevention and safe in both men and women **(Table 3)**.

CONCLUSION

Anogenital warts are the most common sexually transmitted infection with a large incubation period. The infection remains latent even after complete removal of lesions with relapse and recurrences. This carries a significant psychological distress to the patients. The emotional impact on patients can lead to relationship problems with the partner. Proper counseling should be done in patients who are infected with HPV about the infection course and relapse even after complete removal of lesions and counseling should also be done for a healthy sexual behavior. This chapter emphasizes detailed pathogenesis and various modalities for treatment of anogenital warts and also various preventive measures to reduce transmission of infection. Vaccination should be encouraged in age groups of 9–26 years to prevent the occurrence of warts and also the occurrence of cervical and vulvar carcinoma.

REFERENCES

1. Lynde C, Vender R, Bourcier M, Bhatia N. Clinical features of external genital warts. J Cutan Med Surg. 2013;17 Suppl 2:S55-60.
2. zur Hausen H. Human papillomaviruses and their possible role in squamous cell carcinomas. Curr Top Microbiol Immunol. 1977;78:1e30.
3. Fleischer AB Jr, Parrish CA, Glenn R, Feldman SR. Condylomata acuminata (genital warts): patient demographics and treating physicians. Sex Transm Dis. 2001;28(11):643-7.
4. Khopkar US, Rajagopalan M, Chauhan AR, Kothari-Talwar S, Singhal PK, Yee K, et al. Prevalence and burden related to genital warts in India. Viral Immunol. 2018;31(5):346-51.
5. Winer RL, Lee SK, Hughes JP, Adam DE, Kiviat NB, Koutsky LA. Genital human papillomavirus

infection: incidence and risk factors in a cohort of female university students. Am J Epidemiol. 2003;157(3):218-26.
6. Scheinfeld N, Lehman DS. An evidence-based review of medical and surgical treatments of genital warts. Dermatol Online J. 2006;12(3):5.
7. Yang R, Day PM, Yutzy WH 4th, Lin KY, Hung CF, Roden RB. Cell surface-binding motifs of L2 that facilitate papillomavirus infection. J Virol. 2003 Mar;77(6):3531-41.
8. Koutsky L. Epidemiology of genital human papillomavirus infection. Am J Med. 1997;102(5A):3-8.
9. Bouvard V, Baan R, Straif K, Grosse Y, Secretan B, El Ghissassi F, et al. A review of human carcinogens–part B: biological agents. Lancet Oncol. 2009;10:321-322.
10. Dițescu D, Istrate-Ofițeru AM, Roșu GC, Iovan L, Liliac IM, Zorilă GL, et al. Clinical and pathological aspects of condyloma acuminatum - review of literature and case presentation. Rom J Morphol Embryol. 2021;62(2):369-83.
11. Yanofsky VR, Patel RV, Goldenberg G. Genital warts: A comprehensive review. J Clin Aesthet Dermatol. 2012;5(6):25-36.
12. Mougin C, Dalstein V, Prétet JL, Gay C, Schaal JP, Riethmuller D. Epidemiology of cervical papillomavirus infections. Recent knowledge. Presse Med. 2001;30(20):1017-23.
13. Sanclemente G, Gill DK. Human papillomavirus molecular biology and pathogenesis. J Eur Acad Dermatol Venereol. 2002;16(3):231-40.
14. British Association for Sexual Health and HIV (BASHH). (2015). UK National Guidelines on the Management of Anogenital Warts 2015. Clinical Effectiveness Group, BASHH. [online] Available from https://www.bashhguidelines.org/media/1075/uk-national-guidelineon-warts-2015-final.pdf [Last accessed June, 2025].
15. Lawrence S, Walzman M, Sheppard S, Natin D. The psychological impact caused by genital warts: has the Department of Health's choice of vaccination missed the opportunity to prevent such morbidity? Int J STD AIDS. 2009;20(10):696-700.
16. Dong H, Shu D, Campbell TM, Frühauf J, Soyer HP, Hofmann-Wellenhof R. Dermatoscopy of genital warts. J Am Acad Dermatol. 2011;64(5):859-64.
17. Leslie SW, Sajjad H, Kumar S. Genital Warts. In: StatPearls [Internet]. Treasure Island (FL): StatPearls Publishing; 2024.

CHAPTER

5

Cutaneous Manifestations of HIV

Suchibrata Das, Kingshuk Chatterjee

INTRODUCTION

Human immunodeficiency virus (HIV) infects human white blood cells to weaken the immune system. HIV transmission happened by sexual contact, sharing intravenous (IV) needles, blood transfusions, during child birth process and breastfeeding. HIV remains a significant global public health challenge, and currently, there is no cure for the infection. With access to effective prevention, accurate diagnosis, comprehensive treatment, and continuous care—including the management of opportunistic infections—HIV is now considered a manageable chronic condition. As a result, individuals living with HIV can lead long, healthy, and fulfilling lives. Cutaneous disorders are diverse and may be the initial signs of HIV-related immunosuppression. For early diagnosis of HIV infection, it is important to recognize HIV-related skin changes.

EPIDEMIOLOGY

The Global HIV and AIDS Epidemic.

CLINICAL FEATURES IN HIV DISEASE

Human immunodeficiency virus is one of the world's most serious public health challenges. The **Figure 1** outlines the current status of the global HIV and AIDS epidemic, with the situation in India remaining particularly concerning.

Although the adult HIV prevalence rate of 0.20% in 2023 is relatively low, the HIV burden is substantially high in India, with an estimated 25.44 lakh people living with HIV (PLHIV) in the same year. Women are notably affected, with postadolescents and adults aged 15 years and above accounting for 44% (approximately 11.22 lakh) of the total PLHIV population. Children represented nearly 3% (around 0.63 lakh) of the total cases.[1]

VIROLOGY

The HIV belongs to the Retroviridae family and the *Lentivirus* genus. It has two main subtypes—(1) HIV-1 and (2) HIV-2. HIV-1 is the most common subtype and is primarily responsible for AIDS cases worldwide. In contrast, HIV-2 is much less common and is mainly found in West Africa HIV-1 and HIV-2 particles comprise a lipid envelope, contains glycoproteins, including gp120 and gp41, which are essential for binding to host cells inside the membrane there is capsid (core), which is made up of p24 protein, two copies of single-stranded RNA (ssRNA), reverse transcriptase, integrase, and protease—needed for replication.

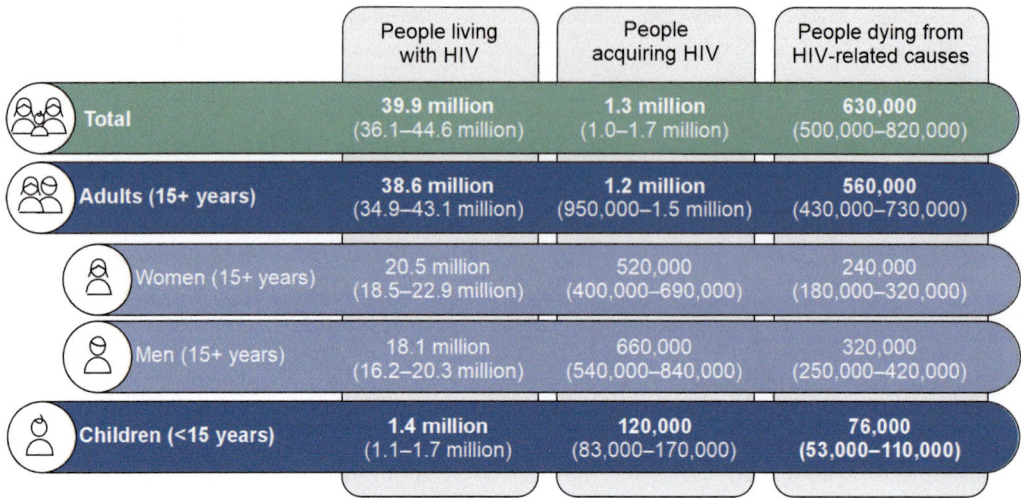

FIG. 1: Summary of global human immunodeficiency virus (HIV) epidemic 2023.
Source: UNAIDS/WHO estimates, 2024.

PATHOGENESIS

CD4+ Th cells are primary target of HIV. This suppression weakens the immune system. Any cell that expresses CD4 and appropriate coreceptor such as CCR5, CXCR4 on its surface may be infected by HIV. If HIV-infected patients remain untreated, they eventually progress to AIDS. HIV compromises the immune system, impairing its ability to defend against infections. As a result, individuals often succumb to opportunistic infections

STAGES

The HIV infection was classified by CDC into three categories, which are as follows:[2]
- *Category A*: Asymptomatic HIV infection without a history of symptoms or AIDS-defining conditions
- *Category B*: HIV infection with symptoms that are directly attributable to HIV infection (or a defect in T-cell-mediated immunity) or that are complicated by HIV infection.
- *Category C*: HIV infection with AIDS—defining opportunistic infections

There are further subdivisions of these three categories according to the basis of the CD4 T-cell count, as those are follows:
1. $>500/\mu L$: Categories A1, B1, and C1
2. $200-400/\mu L$: Categories A2, B2, and C2
3. $<200/\mu L$: Categories A3, B3, and C3

There are three broad stages of HIV that develop over time—acute HIV, chronic or asymptomatic HIV, and AIDS.[3]

After being infected with HIV, there is gradual deterioration of the immune system and the disease progresses continuously from primary infection to death due to the. Clinically, this progression is marked by a sequence of opportunistic infections and malignancies. Nearly every patient with HIV infection, will develop some form of cutaneous disorder during the course of their disease. A wide range of mucocutaneous manifestations may be associated with HIV/AIDS—either as a direct consequence of the virus, due to opportunistic infections, or as side effects of antiretroviral therapy (ART). While some skin conditions are uniquely associated with HIV, many are common dermatologic disorders that present with increased severity, atypical features, or resistance to standard treatments in HIV-infected individuals **(Table 1)**.

TABLE 1: Prevalence of specific mucocutaneous disorders in relationship with CD4+ cell count.[2,4]

CD4+ count (cells/mm^3)	Mucocutaneous disorders	No. of affected patients, n (%)	Mean CD4+ ± SD
<50 (59)	Cryptococcosis	7 (11.9)	48.3 ± 7
	Dermatophytosis	5 (8.5)	
	Ichthyosis	5 (8.5)	
	Kaposi sarcoma	5 (8.5)	
	Erythema multiforme major	5 (8.5)	
	Warts (HPV)	5 (8.5)	
	Herpes simplex	5 (8.5)	
	Oral candidiasis	4 (6.8)	
	Angular stomatitis	4 (6.8)	
	Crusted scabies	3 (5.1)	
	Genital ulcers	3 (5.1)	
	Vaginal candidiasis	3 (5.1)	
	Histoplasmosis	3 (5.1)	
	Acneiform eruptions	2 (3.4)	
50–200 (227)	Papulopuritic itch	73 (32.2)	201.7 ± 111
	Seborrheic dermatitis	27 (12)	
	Ichthyosis	23 (10.1)	
	Kaposi sarcoma	20 (8.8)	
	Dermatophytosis	20 (8.8)	
	Oral candidiasis	18 (7.9)	
	Molluscum contagiosum	16 (7.0)	
	Warts (HPV)	11 (4.8)	
	Erythema multiforme major	9 (4.0)	
	Leprosy	7 (3.1)	
	Psoriasis	3 (1.3)	
200–500 (160)	Seborrheic dermatitis	69 (43.1)	433.2 ± 181
	Dermatophytosis	40 (25)	
	Herpes zoster	14 (8.8)	
	Staphylococcal infections	9 (5.6)	
	Secondary syphilis	9 (5.6)	
	Scabies	5 (3.1)	
	Herpes simplex	3 (1.9)	
	Idiopathic pruritus	11 (6.9)	
>500 (9)	Xerosis	4 (44.4)	503.1 ± 232
	Seborrheic dermatitis	3 (33.3)	
	Scabies	2 (22.2)	

(HPV: human papillomavirus)

Acute HIV Syndrome

Acute retroviral syndrome typically develops 3–6 weeks after initial infection, present with fever (80%), tired or fatigued (78%), malaise (68%), arthralgias (joint pain) (54%), headache (54%), loss of appetite (54%), rash (51%), night sweats (51%), myalgias (pain in muscles) (49%), nausea (49%), diarrhea (46%), fever and rash (46%), pharyngitis (sore throat) (44%), lymphadenopathy (39%), oral ulcers (mouth sores) (37%), stiff neck (34%), weight loss (>5 lb; 2.5 kg) (32%), and other features.[5]

The mucocutaneous eruptions in ARS are distinct, well demarcated, nonpruritic macules, and papules, particularly on clavicular area, but also on upper chest and back, forehead, scalp. Urticaria, pustular, and/or vesicular lesions also present. Noninfectious mucosal ulceration is also a common finding.

Any patient presenting with signs or symptoms resembling influenza, mononucleosis, or other viral syndromes, and who has had sexual exposure to a person with or at risk of HIV infection within the past month, should be evaluated for acute HIV infection. In such cases, acute HIV should be included in the differential diagnosis, and plasma HIV RNA testing should be performed. A diagnosis of HIV should presume when HIB RNA level are ≥200 copies/mL, and it is early to detect and more sensitive than p24 assay.[6]

INFLAMMATORY DERMATOSES

- *Papulopruritic eruption (PPE)*: PPE is the most common cutaneous manifestation in HIV disease. It manifests as chronic, pruritic papules, and sterile pustules, usually presents on the extensor surfaces of the arms, dorsum of hands, trunk, and face sparing palms and soles. PPE usually marker of severe immunosuppression and >80% patients with PPE of HIV-infected individuals have CD4+ cell count < 100 μL/mL. There is waxing and waning and may appear as cutaneous disease in the initial phase of the HIV, when CD4 lymphocyte count is high. The prevalence varying between 11 and 46%, and usually more in less developed countries of the world.[7-10]

- *Seborrheic dermatitis*: It is one of the most common dermatological disorders in patients with HIV (prevalence 20–83%), and has been reported to have distinct clinical and histopathologic features compared to HIV-negative patients. It can appear in any stages of the HIV disease. Frequently occurs early, without any clinical difference with immunocompetent individuals, but in advanced stage of HIV disease, it becomes more diffuse. In addition to face, axillae trunk, and groin may be involved, and may present as erythroderma **(Figs. 2 and 3)**. Treatment includes antihistamines, low-potency steroids, and topical antifungals but widespread disease are more resistant to standard therapy. It is not clear whether ART improves the dermatitis or makes it less refractory to treatment.[11-14]

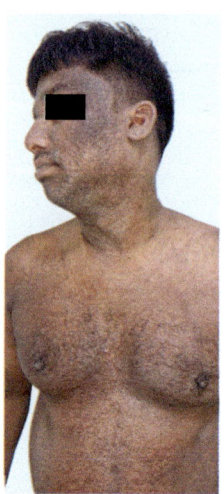

FIG. 2: Seborrheic dermatitis in a HIV-positive patient, on ART, extensive involvement of face and chest.

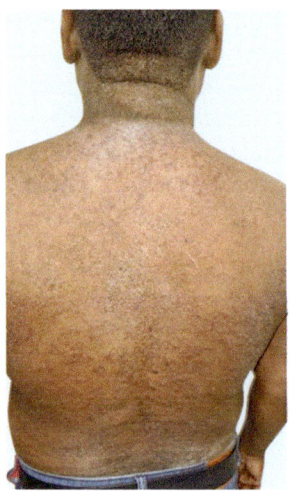

FIG. 3: Involvement of back.

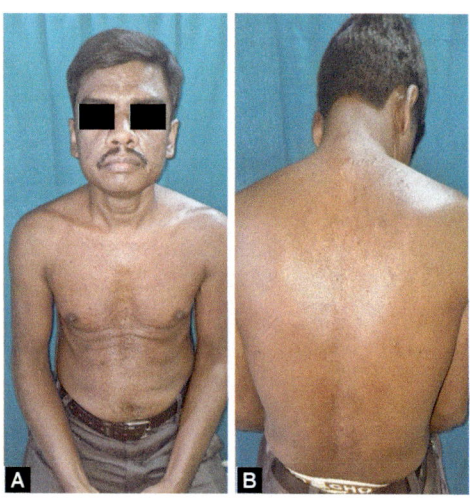

FIGS. 4A AND B: Tiny, erythematous papules, most frequently affecting the shoulders, trunk, upper arms, and forehead.

Psoriasis

The HIV infection may be an independent risk factor for developing psoriasis, and there is no consensus about psoriasis prevalence in AIDS patients but at least as high as in the general population. The most common type is plaque psoriasis, but often progresses to psoriatic erythroderma. Different factors such as the type 1 to type 2 cytokine switch, in human keratinocytes overexpression of HLA-DR, staphylococcal, and streptococcal toxins acts as superantigens, molecular mimicry between HIV-1 env proteins and HLA-DR4 and DR-2, etc., all have significant effect leads to a wider range of presentations such as more exuberant lesions, therapy refractoriness, and frequent relapses. The onset of psoriasis in HIV patients was a predictor of poor prognosis.[15]

Eosinophilic Folliculitis

Defined as an AIDS-defining illness, eosinophilic folliculitis is a noninfectious eosinophilic infiltration of hair follicles. It occurs in persons with advanced HIV disease (CD4+ T cell < 200/μL) and should be viewed as a possible cutaneous sign of immunosuppression, both in children and adults. It manifests as 2–3 mm erythematous, highly pruritic, folliculocentric, wheal-like papules, most frequently affecting the shoulders, trunk, upper arms, neck, and forehead (tends to develop in a symmetrical manner) **(Figs. 4A and B)**. Lesions are extremely pruritic which adversely impacts on quality of life and may cause sleep impairment, distress, and depression. Treatments include oral Itraconazole, oral isotretinoin, phototherapy, permethrin, topical corticosteroids and antihistamines, narrowband ultraviolet B (NBUVB) and ultraviolet A (UVA) with or without psoralen and ART.[16]

Dry Skin

The HIV infection is associated with a number of common dermatological disorders.[2,17] Dry skin (xerosis) is a common skin condition in individuals with HIV, affecting a significant portion of people living with the virus. It is often more prevalent in people with advanced HIV disease and lower CD4 cell counts. Almost 30% HIV-infected individuals had complaints of dry skin or ichthyosis in pre-highly active antiretroviral therapy (HAART) era.[4] Induction of HAART reduces it to a range of 19-28%.[7-9] While dry skin itself is not directly caused by the HIV virus, it is a common manifestation of the weakened immune system associated with HIV, which can make individuals more susceptible to other skin conditions. In the HAART era, there is a decline in infectious dermatological conditions which may a result of a low incidence of opportunistic infections (OI),[9] complaints of dry skin and other noninfectious conditions persist.

HUMAN IMMUNODEFICIENCY VIRUS AND SEXUALLY TRANSMITTED INFECTIONS

Although the spread of HIV is primarily driven by undiagnosed and untreated infections, cofactors—particularly concurrent sexually transmitted infections (STIs)—can significantly increase the efficiency of sexual transmission. STIs do so by either raising an individual's infectiousness or enhancing a partner's susceptibility to HIV. The interaction between HIV and common STIs has been described as "epidemiologic synergy," highlighting how each infection can amplify the transmission and progression of the other.

The STIs have been shown to reversibly increase the concentration of HIV in genital secretions and lower the viral threshold required for transmission. The presence of STIs can lead to mucosal and epithelial disruption, often accompanied by inflammatory cells, thereby increasing the risk of HIV acquisition by up to five times. On the other hand, HIV compromises the immune system, making individuals more vulnerable to acquiring STIs, which may then manifest in more severe or chronic forms.

Systematic reviews have demonstrated that preventing coinfections, including STIs, can lower HIV viral loads and reduce the risk of HIV transmission. For example, treating gonorrhea, chlamydia, and trichomoniasis has been associated with significant reductions in HIV concentrations in semen and vaginal secretions, suggesting that controlling these STIs may decrease HIV transmission efficiency. Notably, treatment of trichomoniasis has specifically been linked to reduced levels of HIV in vaginal secretions.

Furthermore, ART has proven highly effective in suppressing viremia and virtually eliminating HIV transmission among heterosexual couples, reinforcing the importance of "treatment as prevention" (TasP) in global HIV control strategies.[16,18]

Syphilis

Syphilis is often the presenting infection In HIV-infected patients, and HIV alters the natural history of syphilis. Reactivation of treponemal infection becomes more prevalent among patients who are homosexual, bisexual, or IV drug users with AIDS than in the general population, despite presumed adequate treatment in the past.[19,20] Progression of different stages of syphilis appears faster in HIV-infected patients.[20] Patients with advanced HIV infection often have florid and unusual manifestations with extensive or multiple chancres, coexistence of herpes simplex, particularly for those with painful punched out ulcers on their genitalia. In secondary syphilis, the entire skin may be involved with an exaggerated papulosquamous rash as well as granulomatous warty ulcers in the anal region and condyloma lata scattered on their perineum.[19] Tertiary syphilitic lesion such as mucocutaneous gumma may coexists with early and advanced secondary syphilis—suggesting a rapid progression of syphilitic disease within a very short time. Routine serologic tests [venereal disease research laboratory (VDRL) and rapid plasma reagin (RPR)] for syphilis have varied responses and less reliable for active disease. In advanced immunosuppression with CD4 counts near ≤150 cells/mm³, patients of syphilis may present as seronegative. Dark field microscopy and histopathologic examinations may be very useful, particularly in developing countries where facilities for the more precise tests such as fluorescent treponema antibody absorption test and microhemagglutination assay for antibodies to *Treponema pallidum* are not readily available.[19,20] Patients of late disease with HIV-positive treated with benzathine penicillin G 24 million units IM weekly for three doses (USA guideline), some also treat early syphilis with HIV with three doses of such.[20]

Chancroid

The HIV seroconversion is high in chancroid, though it is not a common STI.[21] Chancroid is a significant cofactor in the heterosexual acquisition and transmission of HIV disease with as much as 50- to 300-fold increase of acquisition of HIV infection per each unprotected encounter of vaginal intercourse.[22] The clinical course of chancroid may be altered in HIV disease with prolong incubation period, multiple ulcerating lesions, delayed healing, and poor response or treatment failures.[22,23]

URETHRAL DISCHARGE SYNDROME AND VAGINAL DISCHARGE SYNDROME

Urethral discharge in men is commonly caused by *Neisseria gonorrhoeae*, *Chlamydia trachomatis*, or other nongonococcal and nonchlamydial pathogens, such as *Mycoplasma genitalium* and *Trichomonas vaginalis*. In women, the three most common causes of vaginal discharge are bacterial vaginosis, *T. vaginalis* infection, and *Candida albicans* infection.

In postpubertal women, *N. gonorrhoeae* and *C. trachomatis* typically infect the endocervix rather than the vagina. Consequently, these infections may not always present with noticeable vaginal discharge. When abnormalities occur due to *C. trachomatis* or *N. gonorrhoeae*, they may present as mucus or purulent discharge (mucopus), or as cervical inflammation and friability of the cervical os.

The urethral and vaginal/cervical mucosa contain various immunological mediators capable of responding to HIV and other sexually transmitted pathogens. However, HIV infection itself alters the local immune response and cytokine profile in these tissues, increasing susceptibility to STIs, including those that cause urethral discharge.

Diagnosing and managing urethral discharge syndrome in individuals living with HIV is more complex due to several factors. HIV-positive individuals may experience more severe symptoms, such as increased discharge volume, dysuria (painful urination), and genital irritation. However, due to a weakened immune response, some may have minimal or no symptoms despite a significant underlying infection, complicating early detection. Overlapping symptoms and the possibility of coinfections often necessitate the use of specific diagnostic tools, such as nucleic acid amplification tests (NAATs), to accurately identify the causative pathogens.

The HIV is actively secreted in genital fluids.[24] Men living with HIV who have urethritis show elevated concentrations of HIV in their semen, thereby increasing the risk of transmission. Even among individuals on ART, urethritis can lead to intermittent or breakthrough shedding of HIV in the genital tract, further elevating the potential for transmission.[25]

Although a consistently higher frequency of vulvovaginitis in HIV-positive women has not been definitively established, most studies report a higher prevalence and recurrence of vaginal candidiasis in this population compared to HIV-negative women. Increased *Candida* colonization has been linked to reduced CD4+ T-cell counts—particularly below 200 cells/mm^3—indicating systemic immune compromise.[26]

The HIV infection clearly alters the composition of normal vaginal flora, creating a favorable environment for local infections and STIs. These changes not only promote local HIV replication but may also enhance the sexual transmission of the virus. *Trichomoniasis*, in particular, has been highlighted as a significant coinfection in the context of HIV/AIDS. Effective treatment of *T. vaginalis* is, therefore, an important strategy for HIV prevention.[24-26]

LYMPHOGRANULOMA VENEREUM/BUBO

Lymphogranuloma venereum (LGV) is caused by *C. trachomatis* serovars L1, L2, or L3, causes severe inflammation and invasive infection, in contrast with *C. trachomatis* serovars A—K.

The LGV can be manifested as genital ulcer disease (GUD), lymphadenopathy, or proctocolitis. The clinical findings of proctocolitis are mucoid or hemorrhagic rectal discharge, anal pain, constipation, fever, or tenesmus which can mimic inflammatory bowel disease and proctocolitis is the most common presentation of LGV infection in Europe and North America, due to rectal exposure among men who have sex with men (MSM) or women. LGV among heterosexuals commonly manifested as tender inguinal or femoral lymphadenopathy that is typically unilateral, fluctuant, or suppurative and preceded by a self-limited genital ulcer or papule, occurs at the site of inoculation.[27,28]

There is a higher risk of contracting LGV among people living with HIV. MSM, tested for rectal chlamydia, LGV positivity is significantly higher in HIV-positive individuals (approximately 2.5%) compared to HIV-negative individuals (ranging from 0.12 to 0.33%).[29]

Interestingly, the proportion of LGV diagnoses among HIV-negative or HIV-status-unknown MSM increased from 31.4% in 2015 to 58.4% in 2019.[30] This shift may be attributed to increased testing and previous underdiagnosis. Greater access to HIV prevention strategies, such as preexposure prophylaxis (PrEP), among HIV-negative MSM engaging in high-risk sexual behaviors may have contributed to the changing epidemiology and rising LGV incidence in this group.[30]

The LGV can also affect the progression of HIV. In individuals with HIV, a weakened immune system may result in more severe LGV symptoms and complications. Moreover, LGV may increase the risk of HIV transmission due to ulcers and inflammation in the genital area, which facilitate viral entry.

Patients with HIV and LGV coinfection should receive the same treatment regimens as those without HIV. However, prolonged therapy may be necessary, as symptom resolution might be delayed.[27,28]

OPPORTUNISTIC INFECTIONS

Human Papilloma Virus Infection

Human papilloma virus (HPV) is a common virus spread through intimate skin-to-skin contact. Oral, anal, and/or genital warts, caused by low-risk HPV (types 6 and 11), and different kinds of precancers and cancer, such as cervical, vaginal, vulvar, penile, anal, and oropharyngeal caused by High-risk HPV (16, 18, 31, 33, 35, 51, 53, 56, and 58, etc.), both kinds of HPV are more likely to get in HIV-infected patients. HIV-related immunodeficiency (as measured by CD4 counts) is associated with increased prevalence, cumulative incidence, larger lesions and persistence of HPV infection, cytological abnormalities, cervical intraepithelial neoplasia (CIN) 2 and

3, and ICC. Indeed, HIV have an important excess risk of ICC in comparison with the general female population.[31] There are increased risk and rate of HPV acquisition, more frequent carriage of multiple HPV types, more chance of rapid progression to malignancies in persons with HIV, even they are effectively treated with ART.[32] All HIV-infected individuals and specially who have history of HPV infection should be examined annually. Periodic cervical anal cytology by Papanicolaou smear and patients with abnormal cytology should go for High resolution anoscopy/colposcopy with biopsy, directing toward identifying high-grade dysplasia before progression to invasive SCC. Oropharyngeal lesions usually present as pink or white verrucous papules, and sometimes they transform to verrucous carcinoma. Risk factor associations with oral HPV in HIV-negative patients are sexual transmission and local immunity, whereas in HIV-positive patients, oral HPV detection is strongly associated with low CD4+ T-cell counts.[33] HIV-positive individuals are 2.32 times as likely to develop oral cavity or pharyngeal cancers compared to HIV-negative individuals.[34] When compared to the general population, HIV-infected individuals face a significantly higher cancer risk, with the likelihood being as high as 29 times greater for anal cancer, four times greater for penile cancer **(Fig. 5)**, and six times greater for vulvar, vaginal, and cervical cancers. Among HIV-positive patients, the incidence of anal condyloma lesions varies across different groups: 36.5% in MSM, 14.6% in heterosexual men, and 11.3% in women. Notably, the majority (56%) of these cases exhibit dysplasia, with most falling under the category of anal intraepithelial neoplasia (AIN) grades 1 and 2.[34] HPV vaccines in HIV-positive individuals have variable efficacy, some study, on HIV-positive MSM showed no effect, whereas other studies, one in HIV-positive women and one in HIV-positive adolescents showed reduced effectiveness.[35]

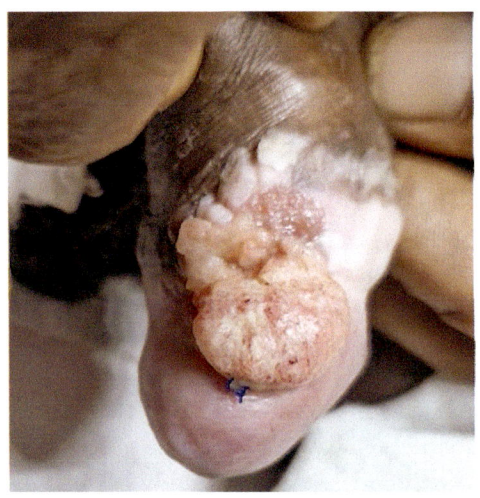

FIG. 5: Penile cancer in HIV-positive patient with genital wart.

Herpes Simplex Virus 1 and 2 Infections

The HIV and herpes simplex virus (HSV) infections cotransmit each other and HSV is one of the most common opportunistic infection in the HIV-infected adults.[36] HSV infection, both primary or reactivated, is known to accelerate HIV progression. HIV acquisition was almost tripled in the presence of prevalent HSV-2 infection among general populations [adjusted RR 2.7, 95% CI 2.2–3.4; number of estimates (N_e) = 22] and was roughly doubled among higher-risk populations.[37] Disrupted mucosal barrier and activated T lymphocytes present at the ulcer base are factors for this increased HIV.

Any site, in addition to anogenital involvement may be affected with these herpes lesion, and in HIV-infected patients it may become chronic, eroded and crusted, or ulcerated, hyperkeratotic, verrucous papules, and nodules.

Chronic herpetic ulcers of >1 month duration is an AIDS defining condition. Lesions respond less with therapy, also recurs.

Chronic herpetic ulcers that last longer than 1 month are considered an AIDS-defining condition. These lesions often respond poorly to treatment and tend to recur.

In the context of HIV-induced immunosuppression, HSV lesions can become atypical and more severe, with potential complications such as dissemination,[4] encephalitis, esophagitis, and resistance to acyclovir.[7,8]

Even when no clinical lesions are present, there can still be excessive viral shedding from mucosal sites. HSV reactivation occurs much more frequently in HIV-positive individuals, with most reactivations being subclinical[9] and localized around the perirectal area. Research suggests that the interaction between HSV and HIV-1 can influence the progression of HIV infection and the development of AIDS. Managing and controlling HSV infections may help slow the progression of HIV.[10]

Varicella Zoster Virus Infection

CD4+ T cells are crucial for fighting off viral infections such as VZV. HIV weakens the immune system by destroying CD4+ T cells, HIV infection can reactivate the varicella-zoster virus (VZV) and cause more severe disease, including disseminated herpes zoster, persistent herpes zoster, chronic and recurrent herpes zoster, and complications such as ophthalmic or neurological issues. The reactivation of VZV infection may occur during the course of HIV infection as an initial indicator of the disease.[35] HIV.gov says that people with HIV are at higher risk for zoster and related complications, and recommends a two-dose series of the shingrix vaccine.

Molluscum Contagiosum

Caused by poxvirus, it is a cutaneous marker of advance HIV disease (CD4+ cell count < 100/μL). In HIV advanced state, lesions of molluscum contagiosum (MC) are larger, confluent and predominantly in face or other

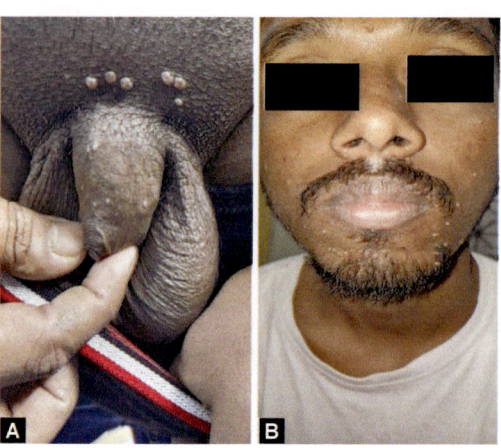

FIGS. 6A AND B: Molluscum contagiosum at multiple site in an young HIV-positive adult.

uncommon areas **(Figs. 6A and B)**. Atypical lesions resembling folliculitis, abscesses, cutaneous horns, verrucous, pruritic or eczematous, condylomas, syringomas, keratoacanthomas, and basal cell carcinomas, also may happen. Sometimes MC may develop as immune reconstitution inflammatory syndrome (IRIS) phenomenon.[38]

Despite advancements in disease management, infections remain a significant source of morbidity in the HIV-infected population. These include fungal, bacterial, viral, and parasitic infections, which often serve as indicators of the level of immunosuppression. Many common infections of general population become more persistent in individuals with HIV infections and also difficult to treat.

FUNGAL INFECTIONS

In comparison to the general population, people living with HIV have a significantly higher risk for fungal infections. These opportunistic fungal infections are superficial fungal infection and deep/systemic fungal infection also. These can cause a range of symptoms and complications, and some can be life-threatening. Superficial fungal infections are common in individuals with HIV, often presenting as seborrheic dermatitis, dermatophyte infections (like tinea), candidiasis, and onychomycosis. Seborrheic dermatitis can be more severe and persistent in HIV-infected individuals. Tinea pedis (athlete's foot), tinea corporis (ringworm), and tinea cruris (jock itch) can be more frequent and severe in HIV patients. These infections can be atypical in presentation, making diagnosis challenging, and may even serve as markers of disease progression.

Candidiasis

Oropharyngeal and esophageal candidiasis are important indicators of immune suppression, commonly seen in individuals with CD4 T lymphocyte (CD4) counts < 200 cells/mm³. *Esophageal candidiasis* typically occurs at lower CD4 counts compared to *oropharyngeal candidiasis*. Oropharyngeal candidiasis usually presents as painless, creamy-white, plaque-like lesions on the buccal mucosa, palate (hard or soft), gingiva, oropharynx, or tongue. In contrast, esophageal candidiasis is commonly associated with retrosternal pain and a burning sensation during swallowing (odynophagia). *C. albicans* is the most frequent causative organism in both conditions; however, non-*C. albicans* species are being reported more frequently, largely due to the increased use of azoles, which create selection pressure.

On the other hand, vulvovaginal candidiasis—whether a single occurrence or recurrent—is common in healthy adults and is not typically associated with HIV infection.

Coccidioidomycosis

It is known as valley fever. In primary cutaneous coccidioidomycosis, the most common presentation is a painless, indurated nodule with ulceration, often on an extremity, but there is risk of causing disseminated coccidioidomycosis, particularly with low CD4+ count produces lesions those may resemble acne, rosacea, or warts, or they may manifest as verrucous plaques.

Histoplasmosis is an opportunistic fungal infection. It is caused by the dimorphic fungus *Histoplasma capsulatum,* the rout of entry is inhalation. It primarily affects immunocompromised individuals, especially those with HIV, and is most commonly seen in patients with CD4 counts < 75 cells/µL.

Cutaneous lesions are observed in up to 17% of patients with disseminated histoplasmosis. These lesions can present as papules, pustules, plaques, ulcers, molluscum-like or wart-like growths, and, rarely, erythema nodosum.[33] Primary cutaneous histoplasmosis is very rare and may appear as nodules, ulcers, abscesses, or lesions resembling MC.[39]

In one case, patients exhibited monomorphic, shiny, erythematous-to-skin-colored papules (0.2 cm × 0.3 cm), and small nodules on the face, upper trunk, and upper limbs. Sometimes, few papules coalesced to form plaques, especially on the eyelids and the nape of the neck, there may be diffuse infiltration, which may involve face and ears.

The infection typically occurs through the direct inoculation of spores via skin and mucous membranes, with thorn pricks being the most common mode of acquiring this form of histoplasmosis.[39]

Bacillary Angiomatosis

Bacillary angiomatosis, caused by two gram negative bacteria, *Bartonella henselae*, or *Bartonella quintana*. It presents as tumor like swelling in the skin and internal organs which is due to neovascular proliferation. Although, bacillary angiomatosis can appear regardless of the immune status of the patient, it usually happens in immunocompromised patients with variable CD4+ count. It presents as a reddish to a purple vascular nodule, as a pinhead to as large as 10 cm in diameter, may ulcerate and bleed. Common site is upper extremities but neck, back, lower extremity, oral mucosa, tongue, oropharynx, nose, penis, and anus may be involved. Histological examination is required for confirmation of diagnosis of bacillary angiomatosis. Detection of immunoglobulin G (IgG) by immunofluorescence assays (IFA), and immune enzyme assays (EIA), have been developed. The drug of choice is macrolide erythromycin/or doxycycline.[40,41]

Other Bacterial Infection: Streptococcal

The HIV-infected patients are at significantly higher risk for community-associated methicillin-resistant *Staphylococcus aureus* (CA-MRSA) infections, both in the community and among hospitalized individuals. HIV-infected patients have a greater prevalence of nasal and extranasal colonization, as well as a higher colonization burden. The perirectal and inguinal areas are the most commonly colonized extranasal sites, and 38.5% of colonized patients had exclusive extranasal colonization.

In terms of factors associated with higher colonization burden, male sex, younger age, and recent incarceration were positively correlated, while hispanic ethnicity was negatively associated.[42]

The most common type of initial skin and soft tissue infection (SSTI) caused by MRSA was an abscess (44%), followed by wound infections (27%) and cellulitis (21%). The initial MRSA infection sites were as follows—lower extremity (28%), buttocks/scrotum (27%), head/face (18%), upper extremity (17%), and trunk (12%). Two patients presented with MRSA SSTIs at multiple body sites, including one case with both head/face and lower extremity infections, and another with infections in both upper and lower extremities.

Risk factors associated with MRSA infection included a CD4 count < 500 cells/mm^3, HIV RNA levels > 400 copies/mL, and injection drug use. 27% of patients developed recurrent MRSA infections, which were associated with risk factors such as hospital admission and a lower CD4 count at the time of the initial infection.[43]

DISORDERS OF OROPHARYNX

If untreated, almost all HIV-infected patients may develop oropharyngeal disorders, and sometimes, it is the first sign of HIV disease. It primarily includes fungal infections, specifically oral candidiasis (thrush), and other opportunistic infections such as herpes simplex and cytomegalovirus (CMV). Oropharyngeal candidiasis, caused by *Candida* species, is a common early sign of HIV and can cause white sores, difficulty swallowing, and pain. Other oral manifestations include oral hairy leukoplakia, Kaposi's sarcoma, gingivitis/periodontitis, sinusitis/rhinosinusitis, mastoiditis, and dental abscesses.[44] ART treatment gives significant improvement oropharyngeal disorders in comparison to untreated patients.

OPPORTUNISTIC NEOPLASMS

Many neoplasms are more likely to develop in HIV-infected people and are considered indicators of AIDS, also known as AIDS-defining cancers. HIV weakens the immune system, making individuals more susceptible to these opportunistic cancers, rather directly caused by HIV infection. Examples of HIV-defining malignancies include Kaposi sarcoma, non-Hodgkin lymphoma, in situ, and invasive cervical cancer.

Other cancers that are more common in people with HIV, though not strictly AIDS-defining, include anal, vulval/vaginal SCC, Hodgkin lymphoma, lung cancer, and cancers of the mouth, throat, liver, and skin. Combination ART is a cornerstone for the treatment of AIDS-related Kaposi's sarcoma, and incidence of other AIDS-related cancers also declined after initiation of ART.[45]

CONCLUSION

The HIV affects the immune system leading to re-activation, atypical presentation and fresh occurrence of multiple cutaneous infections, inflammatory disorders as well as malignancy. Timely diagnosis of these manifestations help to assess the burden of immunodeficiency and timely intervention to reduce morbidity and mortality in AIDS patients.

REFERENCES

1. NACO. (2023). HIV estimation 2023 Technical Report. [online] Available from https://naco.gov.in/sites/default/files/India%20HIV%20Estimates%202023_Technical%20Report_Final_17%20DEC%202024%20%281%29.pdf [Last accessed June, 2025].
2. 1993 revised classification system for HIV infection and expanded surveillance case definition for AIDS among adolescents and adults. MMWR Recomm Rep. 1992;41(RR-17):1-19.
3. National Institutes of Health (NIH) | (.gov). https://hivinfo.nih.gov/understanding-hiv/fact-sheets
4. Nnoruka EN, Chukwuka JC, Anisuiba B. Correlation of mucocutaneous manifestations of HIV/AIDS infection with CD4 counts and disease progression. International Journal of Dermatology, 2007;46(s2):14-8.
5. Hecht FM, Busch MP, Rawal B, Webb M, Rosenberg E, Swanson M, et al. Use of laboratory tests and clinical symptoms for identification of primary HIV infection. AIDS. 2002;16(8):1119-29.
6. Cowan E, Vail RM, Shah SS, Fine SM, McGowan JP, Merrick ST, et al. Diagnosis and Management of Acute HIV Infection. Baltimore (MD): Johns Hopkins University; 2024.
7. Lakshmi SJ, Rao GR, R, S, Rao KA, Prasad PG, et al. Pruritic papular eruptions of HIV: A clinicopathologic and therapeutic study. Indian J Dermatol VenereolLeprol. 2008;74:501-3.
8. Eisman S. Pruritic papular eruptions of HIV-1. Dermatol Clin. 2006;24:449-57.
9. Resneck JS Jr, Van Beek M, Furmanski L, Oyugi J, LeBoit PE, Katabira E. Etiology of pruritic papular eruptions with HIV patients in Uganda. JAMA. 2004;292:2614-21.
10. Bason MM, Berger TG, Nesbit LJ Jr. Pruritic papular eruptions of HIV disease. Int J Dermatol. 1993;32:784-9.
11. Mathes BM, Douglass MC. Seborrheic dermatitis in patients with acquired immunodeficiency syndrome. J Amer Acad of Dermatol. 1985;13:947-51.
12. Forrestel AK, Kovarik CL, Mosam A, Gupta D, Maurer TA, Micheletti RG. (2016). Diffuse HIV-associated seborrheic dermatitis – a case series. Int J STD AIDS. 2016;27(14):1342-5.
13. Kore SD, Kanwar AJ, Vinay K, Wanchu A. Pattern of mucocutaneous manifestations in human immunodeficiency virus-positive patients in North India. Indian J Sex Transm Dis. 2013;34: 19-24.
14. Schaub NA, Drewe J, Sponagel L, Gilli L, Courvoisier S, Gyr N, et al. Is there a relation between risk groups or initial CD4 T cell counts and prevalence of seborrheic dermatitis in HIV-infected patients? Dermatol. 1999;198:126-9.
15. Alpalhão M, Borges-Costa J, Filipe P. Psoriasis in HIV infection: an update. Int J STD AIDS. 2019;30(6):596-604.
16. Cohen MS, Chen YQ, McCauley M, Gamble T, Hosseinipour MC, Kumarasamy N, et al. Antiretroviral therapy for the prevention of HIV-1 transmission. N Engl J Med. 2016;375(9):830-9.
17. Swinkels HM, Nguyen AD, Gulick PG. HIV and AIDS. In: StatPearls. Treasure Island (FL): StatPearls Publishing; 2025.
18. National Academies of Sciences, Engineering, and Medicine; Health and Medicine Division;Board on Population Health and Public Health Practice;Committee on Prevention and Control of Sexually Transmitted Infections in the United States; Crowley JS, Geller AB, Vermund SH. Sexually Transmitted Infections: Adopting a Sexual Health Paradigm. Washington (DC): National Academies Press (US); 2021.
19. Nnoruka EN, Ezeoke AC. Evaluation of syphilis in patients with HIV infection in Nigeria. Trop Med Int Health. 2005;10(1):58-64.
20. Lynn WA, Lightman S. Syphilis and HIV: A dangerous combination. Lancet Infect Dis. 2004;4:456-66
21. Cameron DW, Simonsen JN, D'Costa LJ, Ronald AR, Maitha GM, Gakinya MN, et al. Female to male transmission of HIV-1: Risk factors for seroconversion in men. Lancet. 1989;2:403-7.

22. Ceberry IP, Djeha D, Kacou DE, Aka BR, Yoboue P, Vagamon B, et al. Chronic genital ulceration and HIV infection: 29 cases. Med Trop (Mars). 1999;59:279-82.
23. Mohammed TT, Olumide YM. Chancroid and human immunodeficiency virus infection--a review. Int J Dermatol. 2008;47(1):1-8.
24. Cohen MS, Hoffman IF, Royce RA, Kazembe P, Dyer JR, Daly CC, et al. Reduction of concentration of HIV-1 in semen after treatment of urethritis: implications for prevention of sexual transmission of HIV-1. Lancet. 1997;349:1868-73.
25. Chen JS, Matoga M, Massa C, Tegha G, Ndalama B, Bonongwe N, et al. Effects of Urethritis on Human Immunodeficiency Virus (HIV) in Semen: Implications for HIV Prevention and Cure. Clin Infect Dis. 2021;73(7):e2000-4.
26. Reis Machado J, da Silva MV, Cavellani CL, dos Reis MA, Monteiro ML, Teixeira Vde P, et al. Mucosal Immunity in the Female Genital Tract, HIV/AIDS. Biomed Res Int. 2014;2014:350195.
27. Góes SDS, Fonseca RRS, Avelino MES, Lima SS, Lima MSGA, Laurentino RV, et al. Exposure to Chlamydia trachomatis infection in Individuals who are newly diagnosed with hiv and antiretroviral-naïve from Belém, Northern Brazil. Vaccines (Basel). 2022;10(10):1719.
28. Stoner BP, Cohen SE. Lymphogranuloma venereum 2015: Clinical presentation, diagnosis, and treatment. Clin Infect Dis. 2015;61 Suppl 8:S865-73
29. van Aar F, Kroone MM, de Vries HJ, Götz HM, van Benthem BH. Increasing trends of lymphogranuloma venereum among HIV-negative and asymptomatic men who have sex with men, the Netherlands, 2011 to 2017. Euro Surveill. 2020;25(14):1900377.
30. Prochazka M, Charles H, Allen H, Cole M, Hughes G, Sinka K. Rapid Increase in Lymphogranuloma Venereum among HIV-Negative Men Who Have Sex with Men, England, 2019. Emerg Infect Dis. 2021;27(10):2695-9.
31. Clifford GM, de Vuyst H, Tenet V, Plummer M, Tully S, Franceschi S. Effect of HIV infection on human papillomavirus types causing invasive cervical cancer in Africa. J Acquir Immune Defic Syndr. 2016;73(3):332-9.
32. BHIVA. (2015). British HIV Association Guidelines on the use of vaccines in HIV-positive adults. [online] Available from http://www.bhiva.org/vaccination-guidelines.aspx [Last accessed June, 2025].
33. Muller K, Kazimiroff J, Fatahzadeh M, Smith RV, Wiltz M, Polanco J, et al. Oral human papillomavirus infection and oral lesions in HIV-positive and HIV-negative dental patients. J Infect Dis. 2015;212(5):760-8.
34. Stier EA, Baranoski AS. Human papillomavirus-related diseases in HIV-infected individuals. Curr Opin Oncol. 2008;20(5):541-6.
35. dos Reis HL, Cavalcante FS, dos Santos KR, Passos MR, Ferreira Dde C. Herpes Zoster as a Sign of AIDS and nonadherence to antiretroviral therapy: a case report. Clinics. (Sao Paulo). 2011;66(12):2179-81.
36. Sarna J, Archana N, Eknath T, John M, YS. Protean manifestations of herpes infection in AIDS cases. Indian J Sexually Transmit Dis AIDS. 2008;29(1): 26-28.
37. Looker KJ, Elmes JAR, Gottlieb SL, Schiffer JT, Vickerman P, Turner KME, Boily MC. Effect of HSV-2 infection on subsequent HIV acquisition: an updated systematic review and meta-analysis. Lancet Infect Dis. 2017;17(12):1303-16.
38. Vora RV, Pilani AP, Kota RK. Extensive Giant Molluscum Contagiosum in a HIV Positive Patient. J Clin Diagn Res. 2015;9(11):WD01-2.
39. Patra S, Nimitha P, Kaul S, Valakkada J, Verma KK, Ramam M, et al. Primary cutaneous histoplasmosis in an immunocompetent patient presenting with severe pruritus. Indian J Dermatol Venereol Leprol. 2018;84:465-8.
40. Akram SM, Anwar MY, Thandra KC, Rawla P. Bacillary angiomatosis. In: StatPearls. Treasure Island (FL): StatPearls Publishing; 2025.
41. Ramírez Ramírez CR, Saavedra S, Ramírez Ronda C. Bacillary angiomatosis: microbiology, histopathology, clinical presentation, diagnosis and management. Bol Asoc Med P R. 1995;87(7-9):140-6.
42. Popovich KJ, Hota B, Aroutcheva A, Kurien L, Patel J, Lyles-Banks R, et al. Community-associated methicillin-resistant Staphylococcus aureus colonization burden in HIV-infected patients. Clin Infect Dis. 2013;56(8):1067-74.
43. Vyas KJ, Shadyab AH, Lin CD, Crum-Cianflone NF. Trends and factors associated with initial and recurrent methicillin-resistant Staphylococcus aureus (MRSA) skin and soft-tissue infections among HIV-infected persons: an 18-year study. J Int Assoc Provid AIDS Care. 2014;13(3):206-13.
44. Surdu AE, Loghin II, Dorobăț VD, Hârtie V, Rusu ȘA, Cecan I, et al. Oropharyngeal Manifestations in Patients with HIV from Northeastern Romania. Medicina. 2025;61:855.
45. Yarchoan R, Uldrick TS. HIV-Associated Cancers and Related Diseases. N Engl J Med. 2018;378(11):1029-41.

CHAPTER
6

Danger of Men Who have Sex with Men, Newer Sexually Transmitted Infections, and Sexual Abuse

Vishal Pal, Deepika Pandhi

INTRODUCTION

Globally, the number of sexually transmitted infections (STIs), such as *Neisseria gonorrhoeae*, *Chlamydia trachomatis*, and *Treponema pallidum*, has been rising from the last two decade and there is a further rise of STIs cases in the post-COVID era.[1] Men who have sex with men (MSM) disproportionately experience higher rates of STIs as compared to general population. *Kothis, Panthis*, and *Hijras* (transgender MSM) in India; Katoey in Thailand; and Sray Sros and Pros Saat in Cambodia are examples of MSM.[2] MSM population, due to their sexual behavior, may be involved in both receptive and insertive anal and oral sex and are at risk for anorectal and oropharyngeal STIs, in addition to the more typical genital STIs. The increasing number of dating apps specifically for MSM, decriminalization of LGBTQ (lesbian, gay, bisexual, transgender, and queer), and easy access to healthcare play a role in rising trend in MSM behavior.[3] Extragenital STIs are usually asymptomatic compared to genital STIs, leading to many cases going undiagnosed and untreated. Among MSM, higher rates of STIs are shown by data from several sub-Saharan African (SSA) countries including chlamydia (26% in Kenya and 7.5% in Tanzania), gonorrhea (26% in Kenya and 14.4% in Tanzania), syphilis (12.3% in Malawi and 9% in Uganda), *Mycoplasma genitalium* (36.8% in Nigeria), and trichomoniasis (9% in South Africa).[4] An Indian study with a study duration of 17 years found that there is more than four times increase in number of STIs from Phase I (2003–2007) to Phase IV (2016–2019). They found syphilis was the most prevalent STI at 41.8%, followed by condyloma acuminata at 13.6%.[3]

Nearly 40 years after HIV was first identified in MSM in USA, the global community is witnessing the resurgence and emergence of new HIV epidemics in this population. The approximate median HIV prevalence among MSM ranges from 5% (South-East Asia) to 12.6% (Eastern and Southern Africa). In 2019, 44% of new HIV infections in Asia-Pacific region occurred among MSM. Globally, the likelihood of contracting HIV is 26 times higher for MSM compared to the general population. Moreover, MSM populations have relatively high rates of hepatitis C virus (HCV) prevalence and incidence, specifically among MSM living with HIV and MSM using pre-exposure prophylaxis (PrEP). A global review revealed that the pooled HCV prevalence among HIV-positive MSM was 6.3%, whereas it was 1.5% in HIV-negative MSM. Globally, syphilis is highly prevalent among MSM. In 2019, syphilis affected an average of 11.8% of MSM (ranging from 5.2 to 19.6%) in 11 out of 25 reporting countries, with prevalence higher than 10% was reported from 7 of these countries. Untreated syphilis can result in severe complications in one-fourth of infected individuals who are undiagnosed and do not receive treatment. These complications can be serious and even potentially life-threatening, and they may also elevate the risk of acquiring and transmitting HIV.[5-7]

NEWER SEXUALLY TRANSMITTED INFECTIONS

Increased international travel, social media uses, and unrestricted movement post COVID increase the number of existing STIs and emergence of newer STIs. **Box 1** includes the newer STIs in MSM population. A brief discussion of the individual infection is provided here.

Shigella flexneri

The first case of *Shigella flexneri* transmitted through the sexual route (anal and/or oral) was reported in MSM in the late 1970s. *Shigella* causes shigellosis, a severe gastroenteritis, causing dysentery especially in children. *S. flexneri* is important among other four species because of higher mortality rate. *Shigella* infections are generally considered to be short-lived; however, evidence from serial isolations shows the presence of the same serotype in MSM over a 2-year period, suggesting that MSM acts as a reservoir for the persistence and reinfection cycle of *Shigella*. A study from San Francisco observed that direct oral–anal sexual contact in MSM confers the highest risk and HIV infection further increases the host susceptibility. Apart from the rising infection, another problem is azithromycin and ciprofloxacin multidrug-resistant (MDR) *S. flexneri*. Over the past 5 years, transmission of MDR *S. flexneri* strains through sexual contact among MSM has risen in Australia, Europe, North America, and Asia.[8,9]

Lymphogranuloma Venereum

It is caused by the bacteria *Chlamydia trachomatis*, presents with ulceration of anogenital area. Lymphogranuloma venereum (LGV) infection can present as severe proctitis, proctocolitis, rectal bleeding, ulceration, and tenesmus. Untreated rectal involvement of LGV, especially among MSM, can lead to complications such as colorectal strictures and fistulae. The first infection of LGV in MSM was found in USA in the year 1980. In India, between 2011 and 2019, number of LGV cases rose from 4.5 to 18.3%, primarily among patients visiting the HIV clinic. Apart from HIV, LGV also increases the risk of transmission of hepatitis and syphilis. Approximately 27–43% of rectal LGV cases are asymptomatic and these cases may serve as reservoirs for ongoing transmission of infection. Hence, it is recommended to screen all MSM who have receptive anal sex during the past 6 months.[8,10]

Entamoeba histolytica

Entamoeba histolytica is cause of the amebic dysentery especially in developing and tropical countries with poor hygiene. *Entamoeba* infection ranges from asymptomatic infection to invasive intestinal or extraintestinal disease. It is transmitted by consuming water or food contaminated

---

BOX 1: Newer STIs in MSM population.
- *Shigella flexneri*
- *Mycoplasma genitalium*
- *Neisseria meningitidis*
- Methicillin-resistant *Staphylococcus aureus* (MRSA)
- Hepatitis C
- Ebola
- Zika
- Monkeypox

(MSM: men who have sex with men; STIs: sexually transmitted infections)

with *E. histolytica* cysts. Studies conducted in Australia, Japan, Korea, and Taiwan showed sexual transmission of *E. histolytica* through oral–anal sex and prevalence of *E. histolytica* is higher among MSM including both HIV-negative and HIV-positive groups. Recent outbreak from North America and certain areas of Europe raised concerns on a global scale.[11]

Hepatitis A Virus

It is transmitted through anal/oral route and causes acute liver disease. The first case of hepatitis A virus (HAV) transmitted sexually was identified in USA during the 1980s in MSM. Among HIV-positive MSM in Asian countries, seroprevalence ranged from 15.1 to 50.5% and was associated with increasing age. Recently, outbreaks of 1,400 HAV cases among HIV-positive MSM were reported across 16 European countries from 2016 to 2017. Various studies based on seroprevalence conducted in different part of India, such as Eastern India, Punjab, and Delhi, found that the MSM community had a high endemicity of HAV. A significant proportion of HIV-positive MSM, particularly young sexually active MSM from developed countries, are vulnerable to the infection. Immunization of HIV-positive MSM is important to prevent hepatitis A.[7,12]

Neisseria meningitidis

It causes life-threatening invasive infections that manifest as meningitis and/or septicemia. Meningococci are primarily spread through respiratory droplets and colonize the nasopharynx; however, studies from Berlin and France reported clusters of invasive meningococcal infection among MSM. Reference laboratories in France and Germany discovered the identical genotype C:P1.5–1,10–8:F3-6:cc11:ET-15 in cases of urethritis/proctitis. It suggests that meningococci may co-colonize the urogenital tract with gonococci and this could be due to oral–genital sexual contact. A study by Johnson et al. conducted from 2011 to 2015 found that the incidence of *N. meningitidis* urethritis rose from 2.78 to 8.93%, particularly among male patients.[13,14]

Mycoplasma genitalium

It causes nongonococcal urethritis in men, and estimates suggest that *Mycoplasma genitalium* is responsible for >25% of cases of nongonococcal urethritis. A meta-analysis by Latimer et al. found prevalence of *M. genitalium* in MSM ranged from 0 to 29.9%, with estimates of 6.2% at the rectum, 5.0% in the urethra, and 1.0% in the pharynx. They also found that *M. genitalium* was more prevalent in MSM with urethritis and proctitis as compared to asymptomatic MSM and the prevalence of urethral and rectal *M. genitalium* was more in MSM with HIV infection.[8,15]

Methicillin-resistant *Staphylococcus aureus*

Staphylococcus aureus causes skin and soft tissue infections. Nasal carriage is a significant factor in the epidemiology of this infection and approximately 20% of people are persistent carriers of *S. aureus* in their nasal passages. Methicillin-resistant *Staphylococcus aureus* (MRSA) strain shows resistance to methicillin and all β-lactam antibiotics except the fifth-generation cephalosporin, ceftaroline. A study conducted by Joore et al. in 2013 with 213 MSM found that 12% of perineal sample and 10% sample from glans penis had *S. aureus* colonization (including MSSA and MRSA); however, only two MSM had MRSA isolated from the perianal area. MSM with and without anogenital *S. aureus* colonization showed similar patterns in terms of sexual risk behavior, substance abuse, history or diagnosis of STIs, antibiotic exposure, circumcision status, and hygiene routines. Few case reports have suggested the possible transmission of MRSA through oral sex as well. In one of the reports, a 22-year-old immunocompetent male acquired MRSA through vaginal contact (oral sex). MRSA may contribute to impaired fertility in both men and women, highlighting that it is important to promptly treat asymptomatic carriers who participate in high-risk sexual activities to prevent the transmission of MRSA.[16,17]

Ebola Virus

Ebola virus was discovered in 1976 and was followed by outbreak in Democratic Republic of Congo in 1995 and in Uganda in the year 2000 and 2007. Subsequently, there is an increased awareness of "post-Ebola syndrome" which can persist for at least 21 months after the onset of symptoms. After the disappearance of acute Ebola virus disease (EVD) symptoms, the virus is no longer found in the blood; however, the replicating virus has been documented in ocular fluid, rectal fluids, vaginal fluids, and semen. Secondly, development of acute EVD in female sexual partners of male EVD survivors also demonstrates the potential of Ebola as a STI. WHO advised that semen testing for male survivors should start 3 months post-recovery and continue monthly while practicing safe sexual behaviors, such as using condoms or abstaining from sex, until there are two consecutive negative test results. If semen testing is not available, the WHO recommends that men avoid sexual activity for 12 months after recovery. However, viral RNA was detected in a small number of EVD survivors >2 years after recovery. No study till date available regarding Ebola infection in MSM but persistence of viral in semen and rectal fluid. MSM are at higher risk of getting Ebola infection.[18,19]

Zika Virus

This virus is transmitted by two mosquito species *Aedes aegypti* and *Aedes albopictus*. Zika virus (ZIKV) is associated with an increased risk of Guillain–Barré syndrome and adverse fetal outcomes, such as congenital microcephaly and growth restriction. ZIKV was discovered in Uganda in 1947 and WHO designated this a Public Health Emergency of International Concern (PHEIC) on February 1, 2016. The first major Zika outbreak occurred in France in 2013, subsequently, a second outbreak occurred in Brazil. ZIKV has been observed in the semen of infected males several months after symptoms first appear. Persistence of virus in the testes and semen can elevate the risk of ZIKV transmission via the rectal route in MSM. The transmission of ZIKV from an infected man to a sex partner through anal intercourse was reported from Texas in January 2016. An animal study by Martínez et al. found that ZIKV continues to replicate in the testes for at least 21 days post-infection, and semen, pre-ejaculate, or blood (resulting from rectal damage or lacerations) may also play a role in ZIKV transmission through the anorectal route.[20,21]

Monkeypox

It was identified in captive monkeys in 1958, this virus saw its first human case in a child from the Democratic Republic of the Congo in 1970. On July, 23 2022, WHO declared the monkeypox (MPOX) outbreak as a PHEIC. The disease typically presents with a febrile prodrome 5–13 days post-exposure, along with enlarged lymph nodes, fatigue, headache, and myalgia. Outbreak during 2022 unexpectedly has several cases of atypical presentations, including the lack of early symptoms and the appearance of genital skin lesions. Majority of the MPOX cases during 2022 outbreak were detected in MSM who engaged in high-risk sexual behavior. MPOX virus can be detected in semen samples starting from the onset of symptoms and continuing up to 19 days. Specific sexual behaviors among MSM, such as having multiple casual sexual partners, unprotected sex, and chemsex parties, can further enhance the spread of disease.[22,23]

Men who have sex with men all over the world are overburdened by poor mental health. Studies across the globe consistently found that MSM experienced mood and anxiety disorder, alcohol and substance abuse disorder compared to general population. This may often be attributed to sexual abuse or exploitation that happened during childhood period. Therefore, multispecialty management is warranted.

CHILD SEXUAL ABUSE

A government survey in India revealed that 53% of children experience some form of abuse and the children between 5 and 12 year of age are at greater risk. India is home to nearly a quarter of the world's child population and this indicates a large number of children are at risk. Immature parents, poverty, unemployment, marital problems, alcohol abuse, too many children, and drug abuse are the major causes that contribute to child sexual abuse (CSA). Sexual abuse includes forcing, persuading, or enticing anyone under 18 years of age to engage in any form of sexual activity, regardless of their understanding of the consequences. Signs of sexual abuse are described in **Box 2**. Victims of child abuse gone through five conditions of secrecy (abuse happens when victim is alone with the perpetrator), helplessness (occur due to power imbalance), entrapment and accommodation (due to vulnerability of child), and delayed disclosure (child experience embarrassment, shame, guilt, and punishment), all of these together constitute CSA accommodation syndrome.[24-26]

Child sexual abuse includes early sexual encounter, unprotected sexual contact, multiple partners, and involvement in transactional sex. CSA is a key predictor of high-risk sexual behavior later in life, which increases the risk of STIs and HIV. Individuals with a history of CSA often experience psychosocial issues, such as substance use (alcohol and drug), depression,

> **BOX 2: Signs of child sexual abuse.**
> - Having pain, itching bleeding, or bruises in or around the genital area
> - Have difficulty walking or sitting, possibly because of genital or anal pain
> - Suffer from urinary tract infections
> - Be reluctant to take off his/her coat or sweater, even on a hot day, or insist wearing multiple undergarments
> - Demonstrate sexual knowledge, curiosity, or behavior beyond his/her age (obsessive curiosity about sexual matters, for example, or seductive behavior toward peers or adults)
> - They may go back to younger behaviors like wetting the bed and soiling their pants

posttraumatic stress disorder (PTSD), suicidal ideation, intimate partner violence, and sexual coercion. CSA prevalence among MSM ranges from 15.1% in China to 42% in Latin America. An Indian study from 12 different sites found nearly one-fourth (22.4%) of MSM experience CSA, ranging from 8.8% in Delhi to 70.2% in Coimbatore. The prevalence of CSA also varies among different sexual identities. *Kothis* (receptive partner in MSM) often display gender nonconforming appearance and behavior during childhood and adolescence, which increased their vulnerability to being targeted by older boys and men. Double Deckers also manifest feminine characteristics which may also make them more vulnerable as compared to bisexual (men sex with both male and female) and panthis (insertive partner in MSM). 50% of *kothis* and a third of double decker reported CSA which is far lower than bisexual and panthis. Another important finding this study indicated was that many MSM who experienced CSA may not identify it as abuse, even in adulthood, and may instead attribute the experience to their own behavior. For example, MSM who were targeted due to gender nonconformity may develop a sense of responsibility for the abuse they experienced. Indeed, this pattern of self-stigmatization and self-blame is commonly observed among survivors of CSA across different cultural contexts, and it adversely affects their mental health and well-being. Further, recent HIV-related risk behaviors were 21% higher among those who experienced CSA and MSM with a history of CSA exhibited a lifetime rate of HIV-related behaviors or experiences that is twice as high. A systematic review by Sun et al. provides detailed analysis of mental health among MSM in China. MSM had a lifetime prevalence of psychiatric disorders of 35.2%, which is double that of the general Chinese population. Depression was the most researched mental health and moderate-to-severe depressive symptoms have been reported varying from 26.8 to 53.5%. Depression heightens the risk of HIV vulnerability and those who suffer from depressive symptom are involved in inconsistent condom use during anal sex. The most frequent lifetime mental disorder among MSM was anxiety disorders (20.9%). The disorder was higher in MSM living with HIV (21–42%) as compared to HIV negative MSM (12.6–25.6). A meta-analysis including data from USA, Canada, Europe, Australia, and New Zealand concluded that 11% of lesbian, gay, and bisexual (LGB) persons have attempted suicide in their lifetime. HIV status further increases the prevalence of suicidal ideation to as high as 26.0%. Boroughs et al. conducted a study on 162 MSM with CSA history and evaluate the indicators of CSA complexity and mental health, substance use, STIs, and HIV risk among MSM.[27-29] CSA complexity indicators were: CSA by family member, with penetration, with physical injury, with intense fear, and first CSA in adolescence. CSA with physical injury had four times greater odds to be diagnosed with PTSD and three times greater odds in reporting a STI in the past year. CSA with penetration had threefold increased odds of being diagnosed with current PTSD and unprotected anal intercourse. They also had a greater number of casual sexual partners. CSA perpetrated by a family member is linked to 2.6 times greater odds of developing alcohol use disorder and more than twice odds of substance use disorder. CSA with intense fear had maximum (more than five times higher) odds to be diagnosed with PTSD. The first instance of CSA during adolescence was not significantly associated with any adult outcomes. To identify young children of physical abuse with bruising, Pierce et al. had suggested a mnemonic "TEN FACE Sp," which include any bruising over *Torso*, *Ears*, *Neck*, *Frenulum*, *Angle of jaw*, *Cheeks*, *Eyelids* along with *Subconjunctival hemorrhage* and *Patterned bruises* in a child <4 year of age, should raise suspicion of child abuse. This rule has a sensitivity of 97% and a specificity of 87% in predicting abuse. In the year 2012, Indian parliament passed an act "Protection of children from sexual offences" to safeguard children against sexual assault, sexual harassment, using child for pornographic purpose, and trafficking for sexual purposes. The details of the act could be accessed through the link: *https://www.indiacode.nic.in/bitstream/123456789/2079/1/AA2012-32.pdf*.[24,27,30] The management of CSA is given in **Box 3**.

The resurgence of STI is a cause of great concern and we need to focus on the vulnerable groups and institute adequate preventive control measure and ensure timely therapy.

> **BOX 3: Management of a child with sexual abuse.**
>
> - Thorough medical examination and documentation of evidences
> - Treat the injuries
> - Providing prophylaxis for diseases which could be sexually transmitted or offer contraceptives if penetrative sexual assault has occurred
> - Monthly follow-up till 6 months and look for any mental health issues
> - Family counseling
> - Assist the court in the legal proceedings

CONCLUSION

Men who have sex with men continue to experience a higher burden of both traditional and newly recognized STIs, emphasizing the importance of focused public health interventions, ongoing education, and sensitive, inclusive healthcare services. The emergence of infections such as *Mycoplasma genitalium* and *Shigella* underscores the critical need for enhanced diagnostic capabilities and vigilant epidemiological monitoring. While child sexual abuse represents a separate yet deeply concerning issue, it carries significant implications for long-term sexual health, including increased susceptibility to STIs and profound psychological trauma. Addressing these complex and overlapping challenges requires a coordinated, multidisciplinary effort—combining medical care, mental health support, legal advocacy, and preventive education—to ensure comprehensive and compassionate management for all affected individuals.

REFERENCES

1. Minetti C, Rocha M, Duque LM, Meireles P, Correia C, Cordeiro D, et al. Orogenital and anal infection by *Chlamydia trachomatis, Neisseria gonorrhoeae, Mycoplasma genitalium,* and other sexually transmitted infections in men who have sex with men in Lisbon. Int J STD AIDS. 2024;35(5):379-88.
2. de Vries HJ. Sexually transmitted infections in men who have sex with men. Clin Dermatol. 2014;32(2):181-8.
3. Mendiratta V, Meena AK, Verma D. Epidemiology and changing trends of sexually transmitted diseases over the past 17 years in a tertiary care center: A retrospective study. Indian J Sex Transm Dis AIDS. 2023;44(2):152-7.
4. Mwaniki SW, Kaberia PM, Mugo PM, Palanee-Phillips T. Prevalence of five curable sexually transmitted infections and associated risk factors among tertiary student men who have sex with men in Nairobi, Kenya: a respondent-driven sampling survey. Sex Health. 2023;20(2):105-17.
5. World Health Organization. (2024). Global HIV, Hepatitis and STIs Programmes. Men who have sex with men. [online] Available from https://www.who.int/teams/global-hiv-hepatitis-and-stis-programmes/populations/men-who-have-sex-with-men [Last accessed June, 2025].
6. World health organization. (2020). News. WHO-commissioned global systematic review finds high HCV prevalence and incidence among men who have sex with men. [online] Available from https://www.who.int/news/item/17-11-2020-who-commissioned-global-systematic-review-finds-high-hcv-prevalence-and-incidence-among-men-who-have-sex-with-men#:~:text=In%20this%20review%2C%20the%20overall,)%20in%20HIV%2Dnegative%20MSM [Last accessed June, 2025].
7. Chow EPF, Grulich AE, Fairley CK. Epidemiology and prevention of sexually transmitted infections in men who have sex with men at risk of HIV. Lancet HIV. 2019;6(6):e396-e405.
8. Balaji S, Bhargava A, Aggarwal S. Emerging and re-emerging sexually transmitted diseases: A review of epidemiological evidences. Indian J Sex Transm Dis AIDS. 2022;43(1):20-6.
9. Allen H, Mitchell HD, Simms I, Baker KS, Foster K, Hughes G, et al. Evidence for re-infection and persistent carriage of *Shigella* species in adult males reporting domestically acquired infection in England. Clin Microbiol Infect. 2021;27(1):126.e7-e13.
10. Juyal D, Rawre J, Dhawan B. Under diagnosis of the lymphogranuloma venereum serovars in the Indian population. Indian J Med Microbiol. 2019;37(4):595-7.
11. Escolà-Vergé L, Arando M, Vall M, Rovira R, Espasa M, Sulleiro E, et al. Outbreak of intestinal amoebiasis among men who have sex with men, Barcelona (Spain), October 2016 and January 2017. Euro Surveill. 2017;22(30):30581.
12. Lin AW, Sridhar S, Wong KH, Lau SK, Woo PC. Epidemiology of sexually transmitted viral hepatitis in human immunodeficiency virus-positive men who have sex with men in Asia. J Formos Med Assoc. 2015;114(12):1154-61.
13. Taha MK, Claus H, Lappann M, Veyrier FJ, Otto A, Becher D, et al. Evolutionary Events Associated with an Outbreak of Meningococcal Disease

in Men Who Have Sex with Men. PLoS One. 2016;11(5):e0154047.
14. Johnson L, Weberman B, Parker N, Hackert P. *Neisseria meningitidis*: An emerging sexually transmitted infection. Open Forum Infect Dis. 2016;3:1301.
15. Latimer RL, Shilling HS, Vodstrcil LA, Machalek DA, Fairley CK, Chow EPF, et al. Prevalence of *Mycoplasma genitalium* by anatomical site in men who have sex with men: a systematic review and meta-analysis. Sex Transm Infect. 2020;96(8):563-70.
16. Wertheim HF, Melles DC, Vos MC, van Leeuwen W, van Belkum A, Verbrugh HA, et al. The role of nasal carriage in *Staphylococcus aureus* infections. Lancet Infect Dis. 2005;5:751-62.
17. Joore IK, van Rooijen MS, Schim van der Loeff MF, de Neeling AJ, van Dam A, de Vries HJ. Low prevalence of methicillin-resistant *Staphylococcus aureus* among men who have sex with men attending an STI clinic in Amsterdam: a cross-sectional study. BMJ Open. 2013;3(3):e002505.
18. Tompkins K, Brown J, Tozay S, Reeves E, Pewu K, Johnson H, et al. The impact of semen testing for Ebola virus RNA on sexual behavior of male Ebola survivors in Liberia. PLoS Negl Trop Dis. 2020;14(9):e0008556.
19. Abbate JL, Murall CL, Richner H, Althaus CL. Potential Impact of Sexual Transmission on Ebola Virus Epidemiology: Sierra Leone as a Case Study. PLoS Negl Trop Dis. 2016;10(5):e0004676.
20. Martínez LE, Garcia Jr G, Contreras D, Gong D, Sun R, Arumugaswami V. Pathogenesis of Zika virus infection via rectal route. bioRxiv. 2017:128876.
21. Deckard DT, Chung WM, Brooks JT, Smith JC, Woldai S, Hennessey M, et al. Male-to-Male Sexual Transmission of Zika Virus–Texas, January 2016. MMWR Morb Mortal Wkly Rep. 2016;65(14):372-4.
22. Barboza JJ, León-Figueroa DA, Saldaña-Cumpa HM, Valladares-Garrido MJ, Moreno-Ramos E, Sah R, et al. Virus Identification for Monkeypox in Human Seminal Fluid Samples: A Systematic Review. Trop Med Infect Dis. 2023;8(3):173.
23. Acharya A, Kumar N, Singh K, Byrareddy SN. Mpox in MSM: Tackling Stigma, Minimizing Risk Factors, Exploring Pathogenesis, and Treatment Approaches. Biomed J. 2024;48(1):100746.
24. Paul V, Rathaur VK, Bhat NK, Sananganba R, Ittoop AL, Pathania M. Child abuse: A social evil in Indian perspective. J Family Med Prim Care. 2021;10(1):110-5.
25. Weiss KJ, Curcio Alexander J. Sex, lies, and statistics: inferences from the child sexual abuse accommodation syndrome. J Am Acad Psychiatry Law. 2013;41(3):412-20.
26. Dasarraju RK, Anchala K, Raja T, Manoj K, Sowmy MP, Kumar RV. Child abuse and neglect-How to report a case of child (sexual) abuse in India. J Forensic Dent Sci. 2024;15:3-6.
27. Tomori C, McFall AM, Srikrishnan AK, Mehta SH, Nimmagadda N, Anand S, et al. The prevalence and impact of childhood sexual abuse on HIV-risk behaviors among men who have sex with men (MSM) in India. BMC Public Health. 2016;16:784.
28. Sun S, Pachankis JE, Li X, Operario D. Addressing Minority Stress and Mental Health among Men Who Have Sex with Men (MSM) in China. Curr HIV/AIDS Rep. 2020;17(1):35-62.
29. Brown MJ, Osinubi MO, Amoatika D, Haider MR, Kirklewski S, Wilson P, et al. Childhood Sexual Abuse and Compulsive Sexual Behavior Among Men Who Have Sex with Men Newly Diagnosed with HIV. AIDS Behav. 2024;28(10):3421-9.
30. Pierce MC, Kaczor K, Lorenz DJ, Bertocci G, Fingarson AK, Makoroff K, et al. Validation of a Clinical Decision Rule to Predict Abuse in Young Children Based on Bruising Characteristics. JAMA Netw Open. 2021;4(4):e215832.

CHAPTER 7

Genital Vaccines

Farhat Fatima, Satarupa Kumar, Anupam Das

INTRODUCTION

Sexually transmitted infections (STIs) constitute a significant global public health concern, profoundly affecting sexual and reproductive health. It is estimated that approximately 1 million new STIs are acquired daily worldwide.[1] As of 2016, over 500 million individuals aged 15-49 were living with genital herpes.[2] Annually, around 376 million new cases of one of the four major STIs occur: Trichomoniasis (156 million), chlamydia (127 million), gonorrhea (87 million), and syphilis (6.3 million).[1,3]

The World Health Organization (WHO) Global Health Sector Strategy on STIs underscores the critical role of research and innovation in developing tools to alter the course of STI transmission and achieve the 2030 targets.[4] Current primary preventive measures include sex education and the promotion of condom use. While effective, these strategies have demonstrated limited and inconsistent success due to challenges related to acceptance and improper or inconsistent application. Consequently, the strategy advocates for the advancement of novel prevention approaches, such as the development of STI vaccines. Prophylactic vaccines for human papillomavirus (HPV) are already in use. This chapter focuses on HPV vaccines and examines the vaccine requirements and development efforts for other STIs, including gonorrhea, syphilis, genital herpes, chlamydia, and trichomoniasis **(Table 1)**.

HUMAN PAPILLOMA VIRUS

Disease Burden and Unmet Need

Human papillomavirus represents the most prevalent viral infection of the reproductive tract and is the primary etiological agent responsible for anogenital warts, as well as anogenital precancerous and cancerous conditions, including cervical, penile, vulvar, and anal cancers. HPV infections and their associated diseases constitute a significant global public health challenge, with cervical cancer emerging as a particularly critical concern. Cervical cancer ranks as the third most common malignancy among women.[5] In 2018, it was estimated that there were 569,847 new cases of cervical cancer and 311,365 related deaths worldwide.[6]

Approved Vaccines

Human papillomavirus vaccines have demonstrated substantial efficacy in reducing HPV infections and associated diseases. Currently, three HPV vaccines have received approval for use. The first commercially available vaccine was the quadrivalent HPV

TABLE 1: Overview of vaccines in STIs.

Infection	Pathogen	Status
HPV	Human papillomavirus	Available
Hepatitis B	Hepatitis B virus (HBV)	Available
Hepatitis A	Hepatitis A virus (HAV)	Available
Mpox (Monkeypox)	Monkeypox virus (MPXV)	Available (for high-risk groups)
HIV	Human immunodeficiency virus	Phase I–II
Syphilis	*Treponema pallidum*	Preclinical
Gonorrhea	*Neisseria gonorrhoeae*	Phase II
Chlamydia	*Chlamydia trachomatis*	Phase I/II
Trichomoniasis	*Trichomonas vaginalis*	Preclinical
Herpes simplex (HSV)	HSV-1, HSV-2	Phase I/II

vaccine, Gardasil, followed by the bivalent vaccine, Cervarix.[7] Cervarix provides protection against the two most prevalent cancer-causing HPV genotypes, HPV 16 and 18, while Gardasil offers broader protection, targeting HPV 6 and 11, the primary causes of genital warts, in addition to HPV 16 and 18. In 2014, the nine-valent vaccine, Gardasil 9, was approved, extending protection to five additional HPV types and thereby covering approximately 90% of cervical cancer cases.[8]

Future Directions

The currently approved HPV vaccines are prophylactic in nature, meaning they are designed to prevent new infections but are ineffective against pre-existing infections. This limitation underscores the need for therapeutic vaccines, which aim to elicit cell-mediated immunity to target and eliminate established HPV infections. Ongoing research is focused on the development of such therapeutic vaccines.[9] However, as of now, no vaccine has been approved for the treatment of HPV infections or related malignancies. Presently, two candidate vaccines are undergoing evaluation in phase 3 clinical trials: A DNA-based vaccine, VGX-3100, and a bacterial vector vaccine, ADXS11-001 **(Table 2)**.[10]

NEISSERIA GONORRHOEAE

Gonorrhea is an STI caused by the bacterium *Neisseria gonorrhoeae* (gonococcus). In females, it is often asymptomatic but may manifest as vaginal discharge, dysuria, dyspareunia, lower abdominal pain, or rectal discomfort. In contrast, gonorrhea in males is typically symptomatic, presenting with urethral discharge, dysuria, or rectal pain.[13] Additionally, gonorrhea increases the risk of both acquiring and transmitting HIV.[14,15] If left untreated, particularly in asymptomatic cases, or inadequately treated, gonorrhea can result in severe complications, including urogenital tract abscesses and strictures, pelvic inflammatory disease (PID), infertility, adverse pregnancy outcomes, and neonatal complications.

Burden of Disease

The World Health Organization has estimated the global prevalence of gonorrhea to be 0.9% [95% uncertainty interval (UI): 0.7–1.1] in women and 0.7% (95% UI: 0.5–1.1) in men, equating to approximately 30.6 million

TABLE 2: Overview of HPV vaccines.[11]

Vaccine name	Valency/Type	Schedule (ages 9–14)	Schedule (≥15 years or immunocompromised)	Effective against
Gardasil 9	Nonavalent (6, 11, 16, 18, 31, 33, 45, 52, 58)	2 doses: 0, 5–13 months	3 doses: 0, 1–2, 4–6 months	Cervical, vulvar, vaginal, anal cancers (broader oncogenic HPV coverage), genital warts
Gardasil	Quadrivalent (6, 11, 16, 18)	2 doses: 0, 6 months	3 doses: 0, 1–2, 4–6 months	Cervical, vulvar, vaginal, anal cancers, genital warts
Cervarix	Bivalent (16, 18)	2 doses: 0, 5–13 months	3 doses: 0, 1–2, 5–12 months	Cervical cancer
Cervavac (India)[12]	Quadrivalent (6, 11, 16, 18)	2 doses: 0, 6 months	3 doses: 0, 2, 6 months	Cervical cancer, genital warts
Cecolin	Bivalent (16, 18)	2 doses: 0, 6 months	3 doses: 0, 1–2, 5–8 months	Cervical cancer
Walrinvax	Bivalent (16, 18)	2 doses: 0, 6 months (≥5 months interval)	3 doses: 0, 2–3, 6–7 months	Cervical cancer

prevalent cases. The incident rates are estimated at 20 per 1,000 women (95% UI: 27–58) and 42 per 1,000 men (95% UI: 23–69), corresponding to an estimated 86.9 million new cases globally.[1]

Need for a Vaccine

Current control measures for gonorrhea primarily involve primary prevention strategies, such as sex education and condom promotion, and secondary prevention through early diagnosis and antibiotic treatment. However, these approaches have notable limitations. The growing problem of antibiotic resistance in *Neisseria gonorrhoeae* is particularly concerning, posing a significant challenge to effective disease management.[16,17] Given the high global burden of gonorrhea and the rapid emergence of antibiotic-resistant strains, there is an urgent need for the development of a gonococcal vaccine to achieve long-term control of the infection.[18]

Vaccine Development

The development of a gonococcal vaccine has proven to be challenging. Nevertheless, a recent retrospective case-control study in New Zealand revealed reduced rates of gonorrhea diagnosis among individuals who had received the outer membrane vesicle (OMV) meningococcal B vaccine (MeNZB) compared to controls, demonstrating a vaccine efficacy of 31%.[19] This study represents the first indication of the biological feasibility of a gonococcal vaccine. Although the MeNZB vaccine is no longer available, its OMV antigen, along with other antigens such as NHBA, fHbp, and NadA, is incorporated into the licensed 4-component meningococcal serogroup B vaccine, 4CmenB (Bexsero).[20]

Research has shown that the 4CmenB vaccine can induce cross-species protection against *N. gonorrhoeae* in murine models.[21] Additionally, serum from humans immunized with Bexsero has demonstrated the presence of antigonococcal antibodies, suggesting potential efficacy against gonorrhea.[22]

Future Directions

An observational study has recently been initiated to assess the efficacy of the 4CMenB meningococcal vaccine in infant, child, and adolescent immunization programs.[23] Furthermore, a phase 3, randomized, placebo-controlled trial is currently underway to evaluate the vaccine's efficacy specifically in gay and bisexual men, a population at increased risk for gonorrhea.

TREPONEMA PALLIDUM

Burden of Disease

Syphilis is an STI caused by *Treponema pallidum* subsp. *pallidum*, with an estimated global prevalence of 19.9 million cases and an incidence of 6.3 million cases in 2016.[1] Additionally, approximately 1 million pregnant women were reported to have active syphilis in 2016, leading to 661,000 cases of congenital syphilis (corresponding to a rate of 473 per 100,000 live births) and 355,000 adverse pregnancy outcomes.[24]

Need for a Vaccine

Although *T. pallidum* remains highly sensitive to penicillin and has not developed resistance, syphilis persists as a global health concern. Its continued prevalence significantly affects sexual and reproductive health, as well as neonatal health due to the risk of congenital syphilis. This underscores the urgent need for supplementary preventive measures, such as vaccines, to complement existing strategies for syphilis control.

Vaccine Development

The development of a syphilis vaccine has been hindered by limited basic scientific research, primarily due to the organism's inability to survive outside the mammalian host and the challenges associated with genetically manipulating it, owing to its fragile outer membrane.[25]

The search for an effective syphilis vaccine has proven challenging. A notable study in 1973 by Dr James Miller demonstrated that rabbits inoculated with 60 intravenous doses of γ-irradiated *T. pallidum* over 37 weeks exhibited complete protection against homologous *T. pallidum* infection for at least 1 year. While this study highlighted the potential role of treponemal surface proteins in eliciting protective immunity, its methodology is impractical for human testing.[26] Subsequent immunization attempts with other *T. pallidum* molecules have yielded only partial protection.[27-29]

Future Directions

Advancing syphilis vaccine development requires further research to identify key proteins on *T. pallidum* that can serve as effective vaccine targets. A successful vaccine should aim to prevent the transmission of the organism by inhibiting the formation of primary chancres and secondary lesions, as well as limiting its dissemination within the host.[30]

Notably, Tp0751, a vascular adhesin derived from *T. pallidum* subsp. *pallidum*, has emerged as a promising vaccine candidate. Animals immunized with Tp0751 exhibited significantly reduced bacterial organ burdens upon *T. pallidum* challenge, and the introduction of lymph nodes from Tp0751-immunized, challenged animals to naïve animals failed to induce infection, indicating sterile protection.[31]

In addition to Tp0751, other promising candidates include Tp0136, an adhesion protein, and Tp0663, an outer membrane protein.[32] Continued research into these and other potential antigens is critical for the development of an effective syphilis vaccine.

TRICHOMONAS VAGINALIS

Disease Burden and Unmet Need

Trichomoniasis, caused by *Trichomonas vaginalis*, is a highly transmissible infection that is often asymptomatic, leading to underdiagnosis. Its impact is often underestimated, especially concerning its association with adverse pregnancy outcomes such as preterm birth and fetal loss, as well as its role in facilitating HIV transmission and acquisition. With an estimated 156 million new cases (15–49 years) globally in 2020,[33] it is the most prevalent curable, nonviral STI. Natural infection with *T. vaginalis* does not confer long-lasting immunity, leaving individuals vulnerable to repeated infections. This is particularly concerning given the rising prevalence of strains resistant to metronidazole, the primary treatment option. Resistance, coupled with therapeutic limitations such as the contraindication of metronidazole during the first trimester of pregnancy—highlights the urgent need for alternative preventive strategies.

Vaccine Candidates

Initial efforts to develop a vaccine against *T. vaginalis* began in the 1960s, when women with persistent trichomoniasis were treated intravaginally with increasing doses of heat-killed parasites. While this approach led to reduction of symptoms in the majority (89%) and parasite clearance in some cases (40%), the method was complex, requiring multiple injections at several sites within the vagina and cervix, and repeated dosing—factors that likely contributed to its discontinuation.[34]

In the 1970s, a different strategy emerged with Solco Trichovac, a vaccine made from heat-inactivated, aberrant *Lactobacillus* strains isolated from infected patients. It was hypothesized that this vaccine worked by generating cross-reactive antibodies. However, subsequent findings revealed minimal antigenic similarity between the lactobacilli strains and *T. vaginalis*, weakening the initial theory behind its mechanism of action.[35]

More recent research has focused on animal models. One promising approach involved subcutaneous immunization of mice with a live, whole-cell *T. vaginalis* vaccine combined with aluminum hydroxide (Alhydrogel), an FDA-approved adjuvant. This regimen, administered at 56 and 28 days prior to exposure, reduced infection rates and promoted faster clearance.[36] Other experimental strategies in murine models have included intranasal delivery of a 62-kDa *T. vaginalis* proteinase[37] and a recombinant α-actinin subunit vaccine.[38]

The latest attempt utilized immunoinformatics to design a protein vaccine based on the linkage of the most antigenic epitopes of three proteins: AP65, AP33, and α-actinin proteins of *T. vaginalis*. This candidate demonstrated strong interactions with toll-like receptors 2 and 4, suggesting potential to stimulate both B-cell and T-cell responses.[39] Despite these advances, no vaccine has yet reached human clinical trials.

Future Directions

Commercial vaccines targeting *Tritrichomonas foetus* (TrichGuard),[40] the protozoan responsible for bovine trichomoniasis, have been successfully implemented to reduce infertility and pregnancy loss in cattle. Given the structural and pathogenic similarities between *T. foetus* and *T. vaginalis*, the development of a human vaccine appears promising.

CHLAMYDIA TRACHOMATIS

Disease Burden and Unmet Need

Genital chlamydia infection is a curable and common STI caused by *Chlamydia trachomatis*. WHO estimates suggest 128.5 million new global cases occurred in 2020 among individuals aged 15–49.[41]

Genital chlamydia infection, responsible for nongonococcal urethritis and cervicitis, is often asymptomatic, increasing the risk of long-term complications, especially in women including chronic pelvic pain (PID), infertility, ectopic pregnancy, and increased susceptibility to HIV. The protective immunity induced by genital chlamydia infection depends on interferon-γ and interleukin-12 producing CD4+ T cells[42] and genital tract tissue-resident memory T cells (Th1/Th17) required for long-term protection.[42,43]

Vaccine Candidates

Early research has focused on live attenuated whole-cell vaccines. Although such approaches showed promising protection against genital *Chlamydia trachomatis* infections in preclinical animal models, their use in humans seems unsafe due to concerns regarding potential reversion to a virulent phenotype and the theoretical risk of triggering autoimmune responses.[44]

Killed or inactivated vaccines have been investigated less frequently, but one notable study by Stary G et al. (2015) demonstrated the induction of tissue-resident memory T cells (T_{RM}) in the uterine mucosa of mice following mucosal immunization with UV-inactivated *C. trachomatis* with a nanoparticle-based adjuvant. Mice lacking the T_{RM} cells exhibited reduced immunity despite having circulating memory T cells.[42] However, while tissue-resident immunity, particularly elicited by mucosal vaccine candidates, may enhance protection, recent evidence suggests that its presence may not be absolutely essential for a successful parenteral vaccine strategy.[45]

Following the identification of the major outer membrane protein (MOMP) as a key immunogenic component of the chlamydial outer membrane, various subunit vaccine candidates based on native or recombinant MOMP have been pursued. Tifrea et al. demonstrated encouraging outcomes in a mouse model wherein immunization with recombinant MOMP from *C. trachomatis* serovar D provided significant protection against vaginal shedding and infertility. However, this protection did not extend to serovar F. These findings suggest that incorporating rMOMP from representatives of the three major immunological groups may be necessary to achieve broad protection against all genital serovars of *C. trachomatis*.[46] Other protein-based antigens under investigation for subunit vaccine development include polymorphic membrane proteins (Pmps), the chlamydial protease-like activity factor (CPAF), and outer membrane complex proteins derived from *Chlamydia muridarum*.[47]

Future Directions and Clinical Trials

DNA-based immunization offers a promising strategy for vaccine development by delivering plasmid DNA encoding selected antigens directly into host cells, enabling in situ expression and subsequent immune activation. In an early notable study, a multisubunit DNA vaccine encoding *C. trachomatis* MOMP and porin B, delivered via recombinant *Vibrio cholerae* ghost particles, effectively cleared infection within 2 weeks of genital challenge in mice.[48] Subsequent DNA vaccine efforts have explored various chlamydial antigens, including vaccines targeting the *pgp3* gene, MOMP alone, and the plasmid-encoded *pORF5* protein.[44] While these approaches have demonstrated immunogenicity and partial protection in preclinical models, efficacy has varied.

A rMOMP-based vaccine, CTH522, comprising immunorepeats from four genital *C. trachomatis* serovars (D, E, F, and G) has been shown to be safe and immunogenic in a first clinical trial of a genital chlamydia vaccine in early-stage healthy volunteers.[49] Another mRNA-based vaccine candidate by a French pharma group (Sanofi) has just been granted a fast-track designation in March 2025, from the FDA for a phase 1/2 trial in humans.[50]

HERPES SIMPLEX VIRUS

Disease Burden and Unmet Need

While herpes simplex virus (HSV)-2 remains the leading cause of genital herpes globally, HSV-1 has become an increasingly important contributor, particularly in high-income countries. Often acquired orally during childhood, HSV-1 is now responsible for a substantial proportion of genital ulcer disease (GUD) cases. In 2020, the estimated global incidence among individuals aged 15–49 years was 16.8 million for genital HSV-1 infections (affecting females and males equally) and 25.6 million for HSV-2 infections, with a higher burden observed among females.[51] Lifelong latency with recurrence, asymptomatic shedding, increased risk of HIV acquisition, and neonatal herpes presents unique public health challenges. An estimated 42.4 million new genital herpes cases and 8.8 billion HSV-related GUD person-days recorded in 2020,[51] underscores the critical need for immunoprophylaxis. Current prevention methods such as antivirals and condoms reduce but do not eliminate transmission, highlighting the gap further.

Vaccine Candidates

Herpes simplex virus vaccine development is focused on (i) prophylactic vaccines aiming to prevent infection in individuals who are HSV seronegative and (ii) therapeutic vaccines intended for those already infected, aiming to reduce viral shedding and recurrence.

Multiple adjuvanted subunit vaccines targeting HSV glycoprotein D2 (gD2), with or without glycoprotein B2 (gB2), have advanced to phase III trials as prophylactic candidates.[52,53] The most notable clinical trial, Herpevac, evaluated an adjuvanted gD2 vaccine in HSV-1 and HSV-2 seronegative women in a double-blind, randomized field study. Vaccine efficacy was significant against HSV-1 GUD after 2–3 immunizations but failed to prevent HSV-2 acquisition.[54] Despite generating strong neutralizing antibody responses, progress in developing prophylactic HSV vaccines has slowed due to the limited overall efficacy observed.[53]

There has been a growing momentum in the development of therapeutic vaccines for HSV-2, with various adjuvants and other platforms.[53] Few candidates have progressed to phase II clinical trials. GEN-003 is a subunit vaccine composed of a truncated form of gD2 and a segment of infected cell protein 4 (ICP4), with the Matrix-M2 adjuvant. Its administration in HSV-2 seropositive individuals, in three intramuscular doses, resulted in a 50% reduction in viral shedding and a 65% reduction in days with genital lesions, with effects sustained for up to 12 months postvaccination.[53,55,56]

Other therapeutic vaccine candidates are based on nucleic acid platforms, which typically require fewer doses. VCL-HB01, an HSV plasmid DNA vaccine formulated with Vaxfectin adjuvant, and COR-1, a gD2 codon-optimized DNA vaccine, have elicited weak immune responses in humans with clinical trials stopped after a phase II study.[53,57]

Future Directions

HSV529 is a replication-defective, live-attenuated HSV-2 vaccine candidate engineered with deletions in the essential replication genes *UL5* and *UL29*. While it demonstrated reduced genital disease severity and decreased viral shedding in animal studies, its phase I clinical trial in both HSV-seronegative and seropositive individuals revealed only modest immunogenicity.[53,58]

Nucleoside-modified mRNA delivered via lipid nanoparticles (LNP) holds significant promise for advancing viral vaccine development. Compared to DNA, protein subunit, and live-attenuated vaccines, it offers notable benefits in terms of safety, efficacy, and production costs. In preclinical studies with guinea pigs, a trivalent nucleoside-modified mRNA-LNP vaccine elicited stronger immune responses and provided greater protection than both the Herpevac formulation and the HSV529 vaccine, making it a strong candidate for future human clinical trials.[58,59]

Other notable candidates using the mRNA technology are BioNtech's BNT163,[60] a prophylactic mRNA-based HSV vaccine candidate targeted against HSV-2 and potentially HSV-1; and Moderna's mRNA-1608, an HSV-2 therapeutic vaccine candidate currently in phase 1/2 clinical trial as of March 2025. The HSV-2 vaccine is also anticipated to offer cross-protection against HSV-1.[61]

REFERENCES

1. Rowley J, Vander Hoorn S, Korenromp E, Low N, Unemo M, Abu-Raddad LJ, et al. Chlamydia, gonorrhoea, trichomoniasis and syphilis: Global prevalence and incidence estimates, 2016. Bull World Health Organ. 2019;97(8):548-62.
2. James C, Harfouche M, Welton NJ, Turner KM, Abu-Raddad LJ, Gottlieb SL, et al. Herpes simplex virus: Global infection prevalence and incidence estimates, 2016. Bull World Health Organ. 2020;98(5):315-29.
3. World Health Organization. (2018). Report on global sexually transmitted infection surveillance 2018. [online] Available from https://www.who.int/publications/i/item/9789241565691 [Last accessed June, 2025].
4. World Health Organization. (2016). Global Health Sector Strategy on Sexually Transmitted Infections 2016-2021 Towards Ending STIs. [online] Available from https://www.who.int/publications/i/item/WHO-RHR-16.09 [Last accessed June, 2025].
5. Formana D, de Martel C, Lacey CJ, Soerjomataram I, Lortet-Tieulent J, Bruni L, et al. Global Burden of Human Papillomavirus and Related Diseases. Vaccine. 2012;30(suppl.5):F12-23.
6. Bray F, Ferlay J, Soerjomataram I, Siegel RL, Torre LA, Jemal A. Global cancer statistics 2018: GLOBOCAN estimates of incidence and mortality worldwide for 36 cancers in 185 countries. CA Cancer J Clin. 2018;68(6):394-424.
7. World Health Organization. Human papillomavirus vaccines: WHO position paper, May 2017-Recommendations. Vaccine. 2017;35(43):5753-5.
8. Yang DY, Bracken K. Update on the new 9-valent vaccine for human papillomavirus prevention. Can Fam Phys. 2016;62(5):399-402.
9. Markowitz LE, Schiller JT. Human Papillomavirus Vaccines. J Infect Dis. 2021;224(12 Suppl 2):S367-78.
10. Chabeda A, Yanez RJR, Lamprecht R, Meyers AE, Rybicki EP, Hitzeroth II. Therapeutic vaccines for high-risk HPV-associated diseases. Papillomavirus Res. 2018;5:46.
11. World Health Organization. Human papillomavirus vaccines: WHO position paper, December 2022. Weekly Epidemiological Record. 2022;97(50):645-72.
12. Serum Institute of India. CERVAVAC® Quadrivalent human papillomavirus (HPV) (types 6, 11, 16, 18) vaccine indications and dosage [Internet]. Pune (India): Serum Institute of India; [cited 2025 Jul 16].
13. Piszczek J, St Jean R, Khaliq Y. Gonorrhea: Treatment update for an increasingly resistant organism. Can Pharm J. 2015;148(2):82-9.
14. Cohen MS, Council OD, Chen JS. Sexually transmitted infections and HIV in the era of antiretroviral treatment and prevention: the biologic basis for epidemiologic synergy. J Int AIDS Soc. 2019;22(S6).
15. Johnson LF, Lewis DA. The effect of genital tract infections on HIV-1 shedding in the genital tract: A systematic review and meta-analysis. Sex Transm Dis. 2008;35(11):946-59.
16. Ayukekbong JA, Ntemgwa M, Atabe AN. The threat of antimicrobial resistance in developing countries: Causes and control strategies. Antimicrob Resist Infect Control. 2017;6(1).
17. Derbie A, Mekonnen D, Woldeamanuel Y, Abebe T. Azithromycin resistant gonococci: A literature review. Antimicrob Resist Infect Control. 2020;9(1).
18. Gottlieb SL, Ndowa F, Hook EW 3rd, Deal C, Bachmann L, Abu-Raddad L, et al. Gonococcal vaccines: Public health value and preferred product characteristics; report of a WHO global stakeholder consultation. Vaccine. 2020;38(28):4362-73.

19. Petousis-Harris H, Paynter J, Morgan J, Saxton P, McArdle B, Goodyear-Smith F, et al. Effectiveness of a group B outer membrane vesicle meningococcal vaccine against gonorrhoea in New Zealand: a retrospective case-control study. Lancet. 2017;390(10102):1603-10.
20. Toneatto D, Pizza M, Masignani V, Rappuoli R. Emerging experience with meningococcal serogroup B protein vaccines. Expert Rev Vaccines. 2017;16(5):433-51.
21. Leduc I, Connolly KL, Begum A, Underwood K, Darnell S, Shafer WM, et al. The serogroup B meningococcal outer membrane vesicle-based vaccine 4CMenB induces cross-species protection against *Neisseria gonorrhoeae*. PLoS Pathog. 2020;16(12).
22. Semchenko EA, Tan A, Borrow R, Seib KL. The Serogroup B Meningococcal Vaccine Bexsero Elicits Antibodies to *Neisseria gonorrhoeae*. Clin Infect Dis. 2019;69(7):1101-11.
23. Marshall HS, Andraweera PH, Wang B, McMillan M, Koehler AP, Lally N, et al. Evaluating the effectiveness of the 4CMenB vaccine against invasive meningococcal disease and gonorrhoea in an infant, child and adolescent program: protocol. Hum Vaccines Immunother. 2021;17(5):1450-4.
24. Korenromp EL, Rowley J, Alonso M, Mello MB, Wijesooriya NS, Mahiané SG, et al. Global burden of maternal and congenital syphilis and associated adverse birth outcomes—Estimates for 2016 and progress since 2012. PLoS One. 2019;14(2):e0211720.
25. LaFond RE, Lukehart SA. Biological basis for syphilis. Clin Microbiol Rev. 2006;19(1):29-49.
26. Miller JN. Immunity in experimental syphilis. V. The immunogenicity of *Treponema pallidum* attenuated by gamma-irradiation. J Immunol. 1967;99(5):1012-6.
27. Morgan CA, Lukehart SA, Van Voorhis WC. Protection against syphilis correlates with specificity of antibodies to the variable regions of *Treponema pallidum* repeat protein K. Infect Immun. 2003;71(10):5605-12.
28. Giacani L, Sambri V, Marangoni A, Cavrini F, Storni E, Donati M, et al. Immunological evaluation and cellular location analysis of the Tprl antigen of *Treponema pallidum* subsp. pallidum. Infect Immun. 2005;73(6):3817-22.
29. Sun ES, Molini BJ, Barrett LK, Centurion-Lara A, Lukehart SA, Van Voorhis WC. Subfamily I *Treponema pallidum* repeat protein family: Sequence variation and immunity. Microbes Infect. 2004;6(8):725-37.
30. Cameron CE. Syphilis Vaccine Development: Requirements, Challenges, and Opportunities. Sex Transm Dis. 2018;45(9S Suppl 1):S17-9.
31. Lithgow KV, Hof R, Wetherell C, Phillips D, Houston S, Cameron CE. A defined syphilis vaccine candidate inhibits dissemination of *Treponema pallidum* subspecies pallidum. Nat Commun. 2017;8:14273.
32. Xu M, Xie Y, Zheng K, Luo H, Tan M, Zhao F, et al. Two Potential Syphilis Vaccine Candidates Inhibit Dissemination of *Treponema pallidum*. Front Immunol. 2021;12:759474.
33. World Health Organization. (2024). Sexually transmitted infections (STIs). [online] Available from https://www.who.int/news-room/fact-sheets/detail/sexually-transmitted-infections-(stis) [Last accessed June, 2025].
34. Aburel E, Zervos G, Titea V, Pana S. Immunological and therapeutic investigations into vaginal trichomoniasis. Rom Med Rev. 1963;7:13-9.
35. Gombosová A, Demes P, Valent M. Immunotherapeutic effect of the lactobacillus vaccine, Solco Trichovac, in trichomoniasis is not mediated by antibodies cross reacting with Trichomonas vaginalis. Genitourin Med. 1986;62:107-10.
36. Smith JD, Garber GE. Trichomonas vaginalis infection induces vaginal CD4 cell infiltration in a mouse model: a vaccine strategy to reduce vaginal infection and HIV transmission. J Infect Dis. 2015;212:285-93.
37. Hernández HM, Figueredo M, Garrido N, Sánchez L, Sarracent J. Intranasal immunisation with a 62 kDa proteinase combined with cholera toxin or CpG adjuvant protects against Trichomonas vaginalis genital tract infections in mice. Int J Parasitol. 2005;35:1333-7.
38. Xie YT, Gao JM, Wu YP, Tang P, Hide G, Lai DH, et al. Recombinant α-actinin subunit antigens of Trichomonas vaginalis as potential vaccine candidates in protecting against trichomoniasis. Parasit Vectors. 2017;10:83.
39. Ghasemi Nezhad F, Karmostaji A, Sarkoohi P, Shahbazi B, Gharibi Z, Negahdari B, et al. Introduction of protein vaccine candidate based on AP65, AP33, and α-actinin proteins against Trichomonas vaginalis parasite: an immunoinformatics design. Parasit Vectors. 2024;17:165.
40. Zoetis Inc. (2024). TrichGuard®. Pretoria (South Africa): Zoetis South Africa. [online] Available from https://www.zoetis.co.za/products/beef-and-feedlot/trichguard.aspx [Last accessed June, 2025].

41. World Health Organization. (2024). Chlamydia. [online] Available from https://www.who.int/news-room/fact-sheets/detail/chlamydia [Last accessed June, 2025].
42. Stary G, Olive A, Radovic-Moreno AF, Gondek D, Alvarez D, Basto PA, et al. A mucosal vaccine against Chlamydia trachomatis generates two waves of protective memory T cells. Science. 2015;348(6241):aaa8205.
43. Morrison SG, Morrison RP. In situ analysis of the evolution of the primary immune response in murine Chlamydia trachomatis genital tract infection. Infect Immun. 2000;68(5):2870-9.
44. Schautteet K, De Clercq E, Vanrompay D. Chlamydia trachomatis vaccine research through the years. Infect Dis Obstet Gynecol. 2011;2011:963513.
45. Nguyen NDNT, Guleed S, Olsen AW, Follmann F, Christensen JP, Dietrich J. Th1/Th17 T cell tissue-resident immunity increases protection, but is not required in a vaccine strategy against genital infection with Chlamydia trachomatis. Front Immunol. 2021;12:790463.
46. Tifrea DF, Pal S, de la Maza LM. A Recombinant Chlamydia trachomatis MOMP Vaccine Elicits Cross-serogroup Protection in Mice Against Vaginal Shedding and Infertility. J Infect Dis. 2020;221(2):191-200.
47. de la Maza LM, Darville TL, Pal S. Chlamydia trachomatis vaccines for genital infections: where are we and how far is there to go? Expert Rev Vaccines. 2021;20(4):421-35.
48. Ifere GO, He Q, Igietseme JU, Ananaba GA, Lyn D, Lubitz W, et al. Immunogenicity and protection against genital Chlamydia infection and its complications by a multisubunit candidate vaccine. J Microbiol Immunol Infect. 2007;40(3):188-200.
49. Abraham S, Juel HB, Bang P, Cheeseman HM, Dohn RB, Cole T, et al. Safety and immunogenicity of the chlamydia vaccine candidate CTH522 adjuvanted with CAF01 liposomes or aluminium hydroxide: a first-in-human, randomised, double-blind, placebo-controlled, phase 1 trial. Lancet Infect Dis. 2019;19(10):1091-100.
50. Sanofi. (2025). Chlamydia vaccine candidate granted fast track designation by the US FDA [press release]. [online]. Available from https://www.sanofi.com/en/media-room/press-releases/2025/2025-03-26-06-00-00-3049326 [Last accessed June, 2025].
51. Harfouche M, AlMukdad S, Alareeki A, Osman AMM, Gottlieb S, Rowley J, et al. Estimated global and regional incidence and prevalence of herpes simplex virus infections and genital ulcer disease in 2020: mathematical modelling analyses. Sex Transm Infect. 2025;101(4):214-23.
52. Corey L, Langenberg AG, Ashley R, Sekulovich RE, Izu AE, Douglas JM Jr, et al. Recombinant glycoprotein vaccine for the prevention of genital HSV-2 infection: two randomized controlled trials. Chiron HSV Vaccine Study Group. JAMA. 1999;282(4):331-40.
53. Gottlieb SL, Johnston C. Future prospects for new vaccines against sexually transmitted infections. Curr Opin Infect Dis. 2017;30(1):77-86.
54. Belshe RB, Leone PA, Bernstein DI, Wald A, Levin MJ, Stapleton JT, et al. Efficacy results of a trial of a herpes simplex vaccine. N Engl J Med. 2012;366:34-43.
55. Flechtner JB, Long D, Larson S, Clemens V, Baccari A, Kien L, et al. Immune responses elicited by the GEN-003 candidate HSV-2 therapeutic vaccine in a randomized controlled dose-ranging phase 1/2a trial. Vaccine. 2016;34:5314-20.
56. Bernstein DI, Wald A, Warren T, Fife K, Tyring S, Lee P, et al. Therapeutic vaccine for Genital herpes simplex virus-2 infection: findings from a randomized trial. J Infect Dis. 2017;215:856-64.
57. Kim HC, Lee HK. Vaccines against genital herpes: where are we? Vaccines (Basel). 2020;8(3):420.
58. Egan K, Hook LM, LaTourette P, Desmond A, Awasthi S, Friedman HM. Vaccines to prevent genital herpes. Transl Res. 2020;220:138-52.
59. Awasthi S, Hook LM, Pardi N, Wang F, Myles A, Cancro MP, et al. Nucleoside-modified mRNA encoding HSV-2 glycoproteins C, D, and E prevents clinical and subclinical genital herpes. Sci Immunol. 2019;4(39):eaaw7083.
60. BioNTech SE. A Phase I, First-in-human, Dose-escalation Trial to Evaluate the Safety, Tolerability and Immunogenicity of BNT163 in Healthy Participants. ClinicalTrials.gov identifier NCT05432583. [online] Available from https://clinicaltrials.gov/study/NCT05432583 [Last accessed June, 2025].
61. Vax-Before-Travel. (2025). mRNA-1608 Herpes Vaccine. [online] Available from https://www.vax-before-travel.com/vaccines/mrna-1608-herpes-vaccine [Last accessed June, 2025].

CHAPTER 8

Sexually Transmitted Infection Control Programs

Abheek Sil, Indrashis Podder

INTRODUCTION

Sexually transmitted infections and reproductive tract infections (RTIs) remain major public health concerns, significantly affecting sexual and reproductive well-being. They contribute to a heightened risk of HIV transmission and are linked to serious complications such as infertility, adverse pregnancy outcomes, and certain cancers. Effective prevention, timely diagnosis, and comprehensive management of STIs/RTIs are thus pivotal in curbing HIV transmission and promoting overall sexual and reproductive health. This chapter emphasizes recent initiatives rolled out under phase V of the National AIDS Control Programme (NACP).

BACKGROUND EVOLUTION OVER THE DECADES

India initiated its formal response to the HIV/AIDS epidemic in 1985 through serosurveillance activities, emphasizing safe blood transfusions and public awareness. A structured approach took shape in 1992 with the inception of the National AIDS and STD Control Programme (NACP).[1] Over five progressive phases, the program has evolved into one of the largest globally **(Fig. 1)**.

- *Phase I (1992–1999)*: Primarily focused on raising awareness and ensuring blood safety
- *Phase II (1999–2006)*: Broadened its scope to include prevention, early detection, and treatment services
- *Phase III (2007–2012)*: Expanded services and introduced decentralized management structures
- *Phase IV (2012–2017)*: Consolidated earlier efforts with increased domestic funding support

An extension of phase IV (2017–2021) brought pivotal reforms, including the enactment of the HIV and AIDS

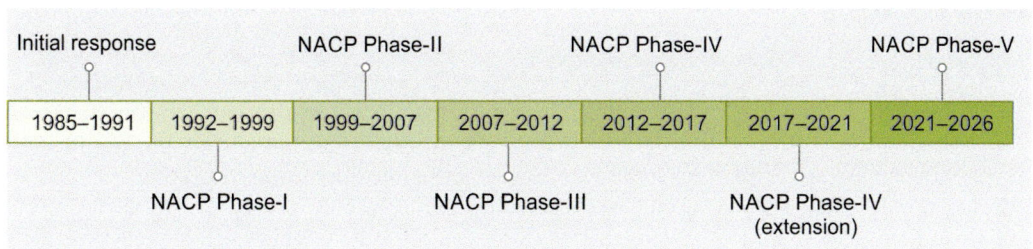

FIG. 1: National AIDS and STD Control Programme (NACP) phases.

(Prevention and Control) Act, 2017, which safeguarded the rights of people living with HIV (PLHIV). That period also marked the introduction of the "Test and Treat" policy, universal viral load monitoring, and "Mission Sampark"—a campaign aimed at re-engaging individuals who had dropped out of treatment.[2]

Need for NACP Phase-V

The formulation of phase V of the National AIDS Control Programme was driven by the necessity for sustained, strategic action to meet India's commitment to ending AIDS as a public health threat by 2030. This phase aligns with key national and global frameworks, including the Fifteenth Finance Commission (2021–26), UNAIDS Global AIDS Strategy 2021–2026, the WHO Global Health Sector Strategies for 2022–2030, and the 2021–24 funding cycle of The Global Fund.[1] The integration of these frameworks ensures that the program remains globally relevant and nationally effective.

The HIV and AIDS (Prevention and Control) Act, 2017

The HIV and AIDS (Prevention and Control) Act, 2017, is a landmark law that safeguards the rights of people affected by HIV **(Table 1)**. It remains important to India's HIV response under NACP Phase-V, serving as a key framework to ensure stigma-free access to comprehensive services.

TABLE 1: Various fields under the scope of the HIV and AIDS Act, 2017.

Employment	Renting/Buying property
Educational institutes	Standing for office (public or private)
Healthcare setting	Insurance provision

Overview of NACP Phase-V

The NACP Phase-V is a centrally sponsored initiative, entirely funded by the Government of India, with a total budget allocation of ₹15,471.94 crore. The program aims to address the HIV and STI epidemics through comprehensive, integrated approaches and by aligning closely with other national health initiatives. The key targets of this phase include:[1]

- Achieving an 80% reduction in new annual HIV infections
- Decreasing AIDS-related mortality by 80%
- Eliminating vertical transmission of HIV and syphilis
- Ensuring universal access to high-quality STI/RTI services
- Eliminate stigma and discrimination related to HIV/AIDS

Objectives

To realize its overarching goals, NACP Phase V focuses on synergizing efforts with related national programs, especially those dealing with comorbidities such as tuberculosis and viral hepatitis.[1-3] The specific objectives include:

- Providing comprehensive prevention coverage for 95% of individuals at risk of HIV
- Ensuring that 95% of PLHIV are aware of their status
- Initiating treatment in 95% of those diagnosed
- Achieving viral suppression in 95% of those on treatment
- Reaching 95% viral suppression among pregnant and breastfeeding women with HIV to eliminate vertical transmission
- Reducing stigma and discrimination experiences to below 10% among PLHIV and key populations

- Offering universal, high-quality STI/RTI services to vulnerable and high-risk populations

The specific objectives of the NACP Phase-V are tabulated in **Table 2**.

95-95-95 Targets (Fig. 2)

India has embraced the UNAIDS vision of ending AIDS as a public health threat by 2030, by adopting the 95-95-95 targets. This strategic goal aims to:
- Ensure that 95% of PLHIV are aware of their HIV status.
- Of those diagnosed, 95% should be on antiretroviral therapy (ART).
- Among those receiving treatment, 95% should achieve viral load suppression.

This cascade underscores the importance of early diagnosis, universal access to treatment, and effective viral control to reduce transmission, improve quality of life, and prolong survival.

Guiding Principles of NACP Phase-V

The success of NACP Phase-V is underpinned by eight key principles that shape the program's design, implementation, and evaluation **(Box 1)**.[1]

Public and Private Sector Collaboration

The NACP Phase-V emphasizes a collaborative approach by building on the existing convergence between national health programs, various ministries, and state-level authorities **(Fig. 3)**. The aim is to enhance the outreach, efficiency, and sustainability of services by fostering synergy across public and private health systems. This involves coordinated planning, service delivery integration, and joint monitoring frameworks to ensure that interventions reach all intended populations effectively.[1]

TABLE 2: NACP Phase-V objectives.

HIV/AIDS prevention and control	STI/RTI prevention and control
• Comprehensive prevention for 95% of individuals at risk of acquiring HIV infection • To ensure that 95% of HIV positive know their sero-status, 95% of those who know their status should be on treatment, and 95% of those who are on treatment should have viral load suppressed • 95% of women (pregnant and breastfeeding) living with HIV should have a suppressed viral load to ensure achievement of elimination of HIV vertical transmission • Experience of stigma and discrimination to be limited to <10% among people living with HIV and key populations	• Universal access to quality STI/RTI services for at-risk and vulnerable populations • Attainment of elimination of vertical transmission of syphilis

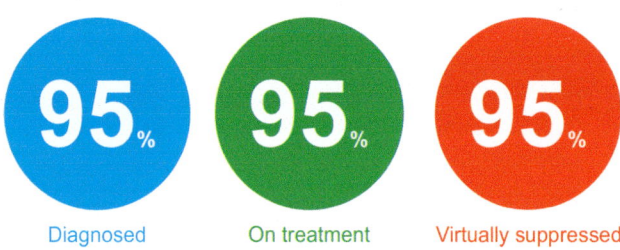

FIG. 2: Schematic representation of 95-95-95 targets.

BOX 1: Guiding principles of NACP Phase-V.

- *Harnessing technology and innovation*: Utilize digital tools and medical advancements to improve outreach and service efficiency. Innovations will be tailored for local relevance and scalability
- *Promoting integration and synergy*: Enhance coordination among different sectors by adopting a single-window service delivery model and establishing robust referral and linkage systems with national health programs
- *Ensuring gender-responsive approaches*: Actively involve women, adolescents, and transgender persons in program design and implementation. Data analysis will be disaggregated by gender to support equitable interventions
- *Centering on community needs*: Deliver person-centered services by linking HIV-related interventions with broader healthcare services, including mental, reproductive, and noncommunicable disease care.
- *Evidence-based planning and monitoring*: Use real-time, granular, and cross-sectional data to guide planning, implementation, course correction, and performance evaluation
- *Decentralized high-impact program management*: Strengthen district-level management through strategies such as DISHA (district Integrated Strategy for HIV/AIDS), with a focus on effective supply chain and resource optimization
- *Partnership enhancement*: Foster collaboration across government departments, civil society organizations, private sector stakeholders, and international partners to expand the program's reach and impact
- *Institutional capacity building*: Strengthen technical infrastructure by empowering existing bodies such as technical resource groups (TRGs) and technical working groups (TWGs) to guide the program with scientific rigor

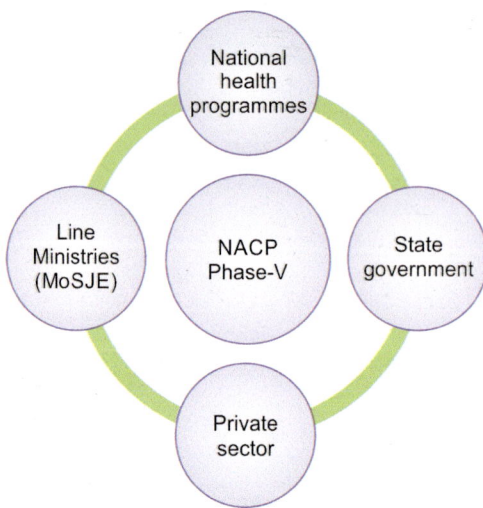

FIG. 3: Various collaborating agencies (public and private) under NACP Phase-V.

Strategies for Goal Implementation[1]

Goal 1: Reduce annual new HIV infections by 80%.	
Strengthening targeted interventions (TIs) and link worker schemes (LWS)	Existing peer-led outreach models such as TIs and LWS are being enhanced to provide integrated services to high-risk groups (HRGs) and other vulnerable groups at physical hotspots **(Table 3)**. This includes the introduction of *dual HIV-syphilis rapid diagnostic kits* to boost early detection and service uptake. The referral and linkage system will be further utilized to identify and record comorbidities in such patients **(Fig. 4)**
Customizing prevention packages by location and population	Evidence-driven and location-specific strategies are promoted to ensure contextual relevance. This includes improved data collection to inform targeted interventions based on local epidemiology
Enhancing population size estimates and intelligence	Efforts are underway to refine population size estimations and gather field-based intelligence using tools such as *programmatic mapping and population size estimation (p-MPSE)* for saturation of services
Expanding harm reduction initiatives for IDUs (injecting drug users)	Key harm reduction programs such as the *needle-syringe exchange program (NSEP)* and *opioid substitution therapy (OST)* are being scaled up in partnership with the Ministry of Social Justice and Empowerment, with linkages to hepatitis services under NVHCP to reduce comorbidity
Reaching incarcerated populations	HIV, TB, and hepatitis services are being integrated into correctional facilities. Additionally, referral systems are set up for inmates' postrelease to ensure continuity of care
Community-based integrated service models	Models like *one-stop centers (OSCs)* **(Box 2 and Flowcharts 1 and 2)** are being piloted and expanded. These community hubs provide bundled services including HIV testing, STI treatment, counseling, and social support, tailored to high-risk populations
Expanding coverage among bridge populations	Bridge populations such as *migrants* and *truckers* are targeted using employer-led models, LWS, and customized TIs. Research will also identify other subgroups under this category to develop specific intervention models
Innovating communication strategies	A fresh communication strategy is being rolled out, leveraging digital platforms (Internet and mobile apps) to engage populations that may not perceive themselves at risk but exhibit risk behaviors
Sampoorna Suraksha Strategy (SSS)	This initiative caters to HIV-negative but at-risk individuals who fall outside traditional TI categories. Using a cyclical and comprehensive service package, SSS ensures that they remain HIV free. Key entry points include *ICTCs, STI clinics, and virtual outreach platforms*
Virtual interventions for online populations	Given the growing use of virtual platforms **(Table 4)** by young people, MSM, and sex workers, new models will engage these groups with online education, risk assessment, and linkage to testing services. The *1097 Toll-Free AIDS Helpline* anchors these efforts
Behavior change campaigns for the general public	Mass media and interpersonal communication strategies are maintained to ensure sustained awareness among the general population. The National Toll-Free AIDS Helpline – 1097 is an important link for service access
Youth-focused programming	Adolescents and young adults are prioritized through peer-led initiatives that promote safe behaviors, STI/HIV education, and early testing

TABLE 3: Classification of high-risk groups.

High-risk groups (HRGs)		
Core population: • Female sex workers (FSW) • Male having sex with men (MSM) • People who inject drugs (PWID) • *Hijra*/Transgenders (H/TGs)	*Bridge population:* • Truckers • Migrants	Prison and other closed settings

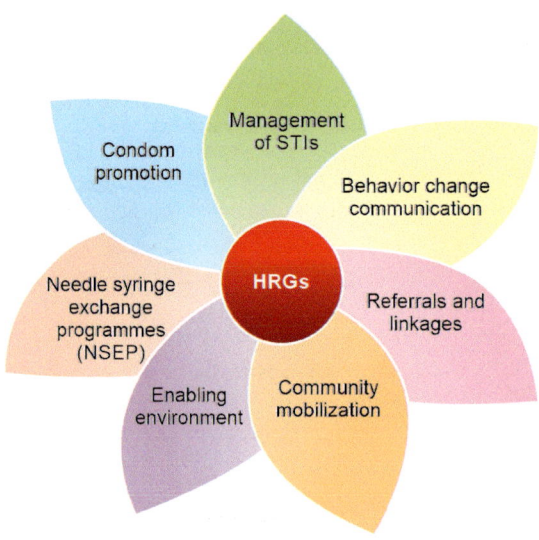

FIG. 4: Targeted interventions in high-risk groups (HRGs).

BOX 2: Overview of one-stop centers.

One-stop centers (OSCs)
- Integrated service delivery model at community settings
- Person-centered and resource-effective approach to deliver integrated HIV prevention services in settings with low-concentrated HIV epidemics
- Community-based centers which are designed to be a single umbrella approach to attract the key and bridge population

Objectives:
- Promote screening and linkage for HIV and other essential health services
- Promote screening and referral to requisite holistic care services
- Ensure completion of referrals/linkages among the different service providers
- Increase access to HIV, other essential health services, and social welfare services
- Increase awareness and reduce stigma and discrimination

Service benefits:
- Adequate infrastructure
- Recreational facilities
- Flexible timings
- Community preferred doctor
- Nonstigmatizing environment
- OSCs will improve general health and well-being by helping them reduce the harm associated with risk behaviors

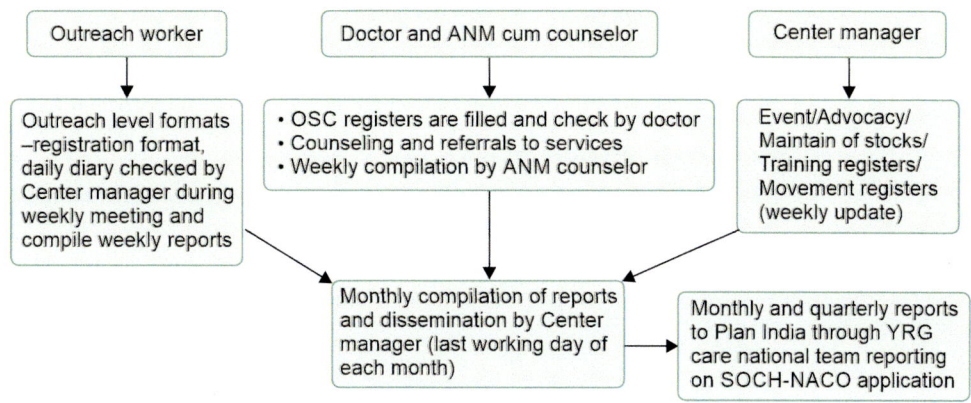

FLOWCHART 1: Flow of services at one-stop centers (OSCs).
(ANM: auxiliary nurse midwife; NACO: National AIDS Control Organization; SOCH: strengthening overall care for HIV beneficiaries)

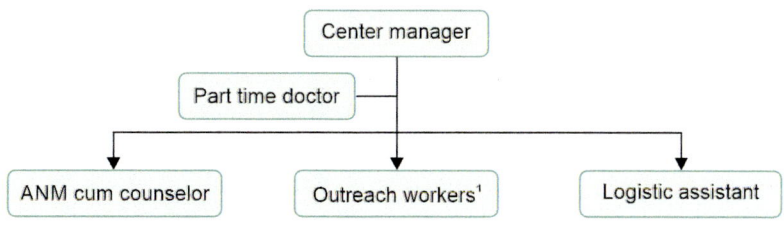

FLOWCHART 2: Staff at one-stop centers (OSCs).

TABLE 4: Virtual interventions under NACP-V.

Featured virtual strategies for HIV care in India	
Virtual DIC, Delhi SACS, FSW/MSM/TG	Risk awareness, prevention, testing, and service linkage
MDACS/HST, ITECH-CDC, young MSM	Risk awareness, prevention, testing, and service linkage
Maharashtra SACS, HRGs (FSW)	Knowledge, awareness, feedback, and planning
Ujwala project—Alliance India, FSW	Prevention, testing, treatment, and care support
Yes4Me—USAID, general, and KPs	Risk assessment, prevention, testing, and service linkage
Safe Masti—Elton John AIDS Foundation, young MSM	Awareness, prevention, and stigma reduction
Virtual outreach, Nagaland, ITECH-CDC, MSM, and TG	Outreach, awareness, HIV testing and treatment services, distribution of commodities

Goal 2: Reduce AIDS-related mortalities by 80%.

Expanding HIV counseling and testing services (HCTS)	HIV testing will continue through a mix of service models—standalone centers, mobile units, and facilities integrated within both public and private healthcare settings. Community-based screening (CBS) models will also be strengthened to improve outreach in hard-to-reach areas
Focused communication to boost testing uptake	Special campaigns will be rolled out targeting adolescents and youth to improve awareness and increase uptake of HIV testing. Platforms such as *Red Ribbon Clubs* and the *Adolescence Education Programme (AEP)* will be actively leveraged
Active case finding and early diagnosis	To enhance the detection of undiagnosed cases, techniques such as *social network testing, index testing*, and *repeat testing for discordant couples* will be implemented. These approaches are expected to increase the efficiency of existing HCTS models
Integrating new testing technologies	The program will generate evidence on innovative testing options such as *HIV self-testing*, enabling informed decisions about scaling these models across diverse populations and regions
Sustaining and scaling up care, support, and treatment (CST) services	The established three-tier CST framework **(Fig. 5)** will continue to serve as the backbone of HIV care. Expansion of ART centers will be undertaken, particularly through public medical colleges and collaboration with private hospitals and laboratories
Improving access to high-quality ART	NACP Phase-V promotes *Dolutegravir-based regimens* as the preferred ART option, due to their superior outcomes in terms of viral suppression, adherence, and tolerability. These regimens will also be introduced for *Postexposure prophylaxis (PEP). Differentiated service delivery models*—such as community-based drug refills and multi-month dispensing—will improve retention and convenience for PLHIV
Rapid ART initiation and management of advanced HIV disease	Timely ART initiation is crucial. Ideally, treatment should begin within 7 days of diagnosis, and same-day initiation will be offered to those ready. Individuals presenting with advanced HIV disease will receive priority for immediate clinical management
Updating clinical guidelines regularly	Treatment protocols will be reviewed and revised based on emerging scientific evidence. Options such as *dual therapy, long-acting injectables*, and *implants* are being evaluated for simplified and more sustainable disease management
Minimizing linkage loss	To prevent drop-offs between diagnosis and treatment, predictive analytics using *machine learning* and centralized data systems will help identify and engage individuals at risk of discontinuation. Customized counseling and follow-up strategies will be applied
Enhancing viral load monitoring	The program will expand *dried blood spot (DBS)* sample collection to improve access to viral load testing. Selected public laboratories will be upgraded for *drug resistance monitoring*, ensuring timely and effective treatment adjustments. **(Fig. 6)**
Integrated service packages for PLHIV and at-risk groups	Holistic service packages—including HIV, TB, STI, hepatitis, and mental health services—will be delivered through integrated referral and linkage systems in collaboration with other health programs
Prioritizing women's health	Women living with HIV will receive focused support, including *reproductive health services, family planning*, and *early infant diagnosis*. Coordination with the *National Health Mission (NHM)* will support this comprehensive care approach

Continued

Continued

Goal 2: Reduce AIDS-related mortalities by 80%.

Enhancing service efficiency through single-window models	Service delivery will be reorganized in selected locations for efficiency. This includes better space utilization, task shifting, and the adoption of IT-enabled systems, backed by focused training and capacity-building of staff **(Flowchart 3)**
Strengthening laboratory quality systems	The quality assurance framework will now go beyond HIV testing to include STI/RTI diagnostics. This involves *proficiency testing, inter-laboratory comparisons*, and *laboratory accreditations*, ensuring high standards across the diagnostic chain

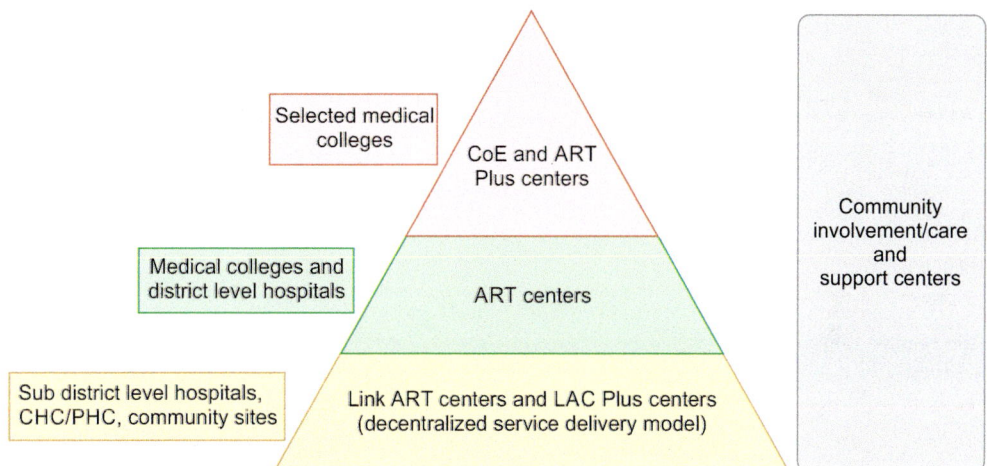

FIG. 5: HIV care, support, and treatment services.
(ART: antiretroviral therapy; CHC: community health center; CoE: center of excellence; PHC: primary health care)

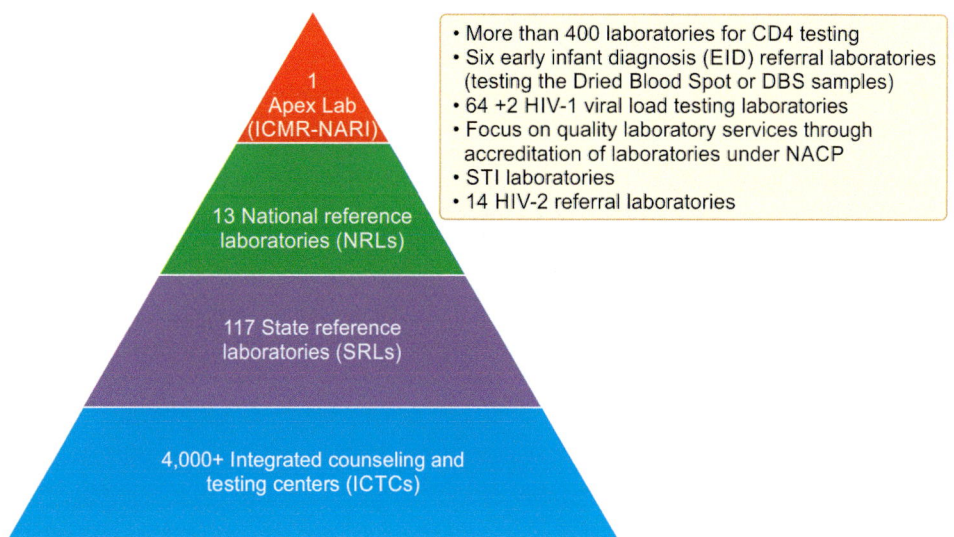

FIG. 6: HIV laboratory services.

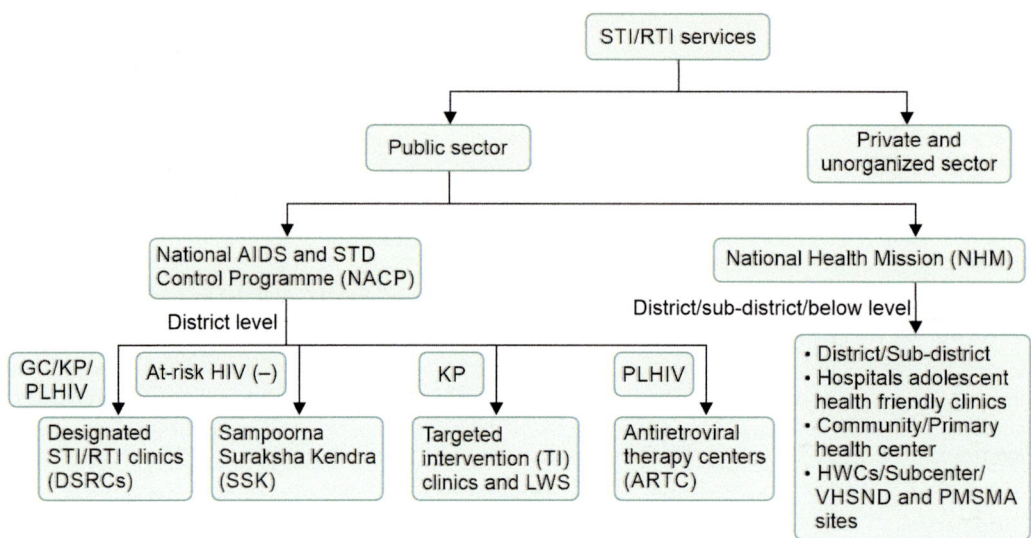

FLOWCHART 3: Sexually transmitted infection (STI) and reproductive tract infection (RTI) services delivery in India.

Goal 3: Eliminate vertical transmission of HIV and syphilis.	
Integrating with NHM for universal antenatal testing	A strategic collaboration with the *National Health Mission (NHM)* facilitates universal HIV and syphilis testing during pregnancy. Prioritized district-level interventions ensure complete coverage, with data from HMIS and RCH portals being integrated into NACP systems for immediate confirmatory testing and linkage to care
Strengthening primary prevention efforts	Awareness campaigns and behavior change interventions focused on safe sexual practices are being scaled up. Adolescents and young women are engaged through joint programs of NHM (e.g., *RKSK*) and NACP (e.g., *Red Ribbon Clubs* and *AEP*) to reduce new infections and associated risks
Rolling out dual test kits	Rapid diagnostic kits capable of simultaneously detecting HIV and syphilis are being deployed at antenatal clinics and labor rooms. This dual testing approach allows for early identification and immediate initiation of treatment, minimizing the window for vertical transmission **(Fig. 7 and Flowchart 4)**
Ensuring linkage to treatment	Not all women who test positive for HIV during antenatal screening reach confirmatory centers or begin ART. To address this gap, targeted outreach, use of digital tools, and structured review mechanisms will be employed to strengthen the continuum of care
Promoting ART adherence among WLHIV	Pregnant and breastfeeding women living with HIV (WLHIV) will receive ongoing counseling and support to achieve sustained viral suppression. Confidential, community-based service delivery models will be scaled up to reduce stigma and improve adherence

Continued

Continued

Goal 3: Eliminate vertical transmission of HIV and syphilis.	
Integrating family planning services	All PLHIV, especially women, will be assessed during their ART center visits for contraceptive needs and referred to family planning services, ensuring informed reproductive choices and preventing unintended pregnancies
Early diagnosis and management of infants	Emphasis will be placed on *early infant diagnosis (EID)* and HIV testing of family members. Identified *children living with HIV (CLHIV)* will be promptly linked to ART services to improve long-term outcomes
Engaging the private sector	Private healthcare providers will be sensitized and engaged in dual elimination efforts. They will be encouraged to offer routine antenatal testing and appropriate treatment (e.g., *benzathine penicillin G* for syphilis-positive pregnant women)
Improving strategic information	Efforts will be made to strengthen data systems for tracking fertility patterns among WLHIV, adherence to ART during and after pregnancy, and identification of HIV-exposed infants. Integrated monitoring using research, epidemiology, and surveillance data will guide program actions
Roadmap for validation of elimination	A structured action plan will be developed using WHO-recommended tools to assess progress and guide interventions toward validated elimination of vertical transmission. This roadmap will include clearly defined milestones and timelines
Enhancing behavior change communication	Social media campaigns and digital outreach will be leveraged for cost-effective dissemination of information. The *National Toll-Free AIDS Helpline (1097)* will support awareness efforts and facilitate service linkages
Sustained youth engagement	Adolescent-focused interventions will promote uptake of HIV-related services through age- and gender-appropriate messaging and delivery platforms, in alignment with national policies

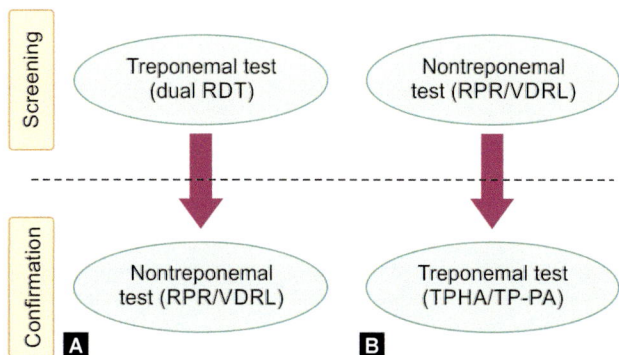

FIGS. 7A AND B: Reverse testing algorithm for syphilis. (A) Reverse algorithm—treponemal antibody testing (e.g., dual RDT); (B) Traditional algorithm—nontreponemal antibody testing (e.g., RPR)-traditional syphilis screening algorithm.

(RDT: rapid diagnostic test; RPR: rapid plasma reagin; TPHA: *Treponema pallidum* hemagglutination assay; TP-PA: *Treponema pallidum* particle agglutination; VDRL: venereal disease research laboratory)

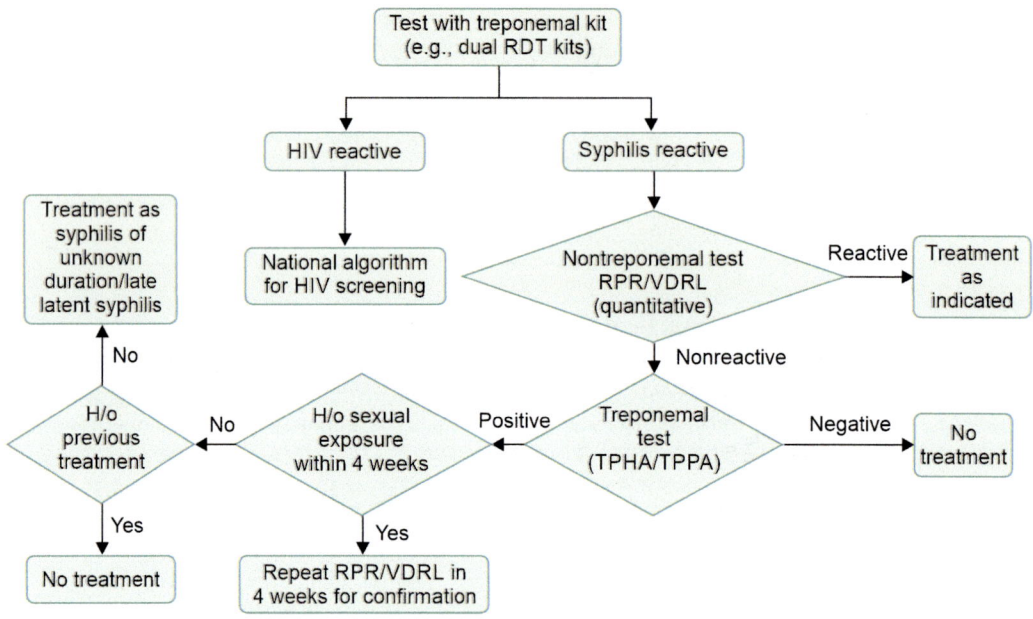

FLOWCHART 4: Reverse treatment algorithm for syphilis.
(TPHA: *Treponema pallidum* hemagglutination assay; TPPA: *Treponema pallidum* particle agglutination)

Goal 4: Promote universal access to quality STI/RTI services to at-risk and vulnerable populations.	
Enhancing strategic information on STIs	Improved data collection, monitoring, and analysis are central to informing STI interventions. The program promotes a multidimensional information ecosystem involving surveillance, research, and evaluation to track trends, identify gaps, and guide responses
Strengthening the designated STI/RTI clinics (DSRC) model	DSRCs will continue to anchor STI/RTI services using a dual setup under the departments of Obstetrics and Gynecology and Dermatology/Venereology. These clinics will also coordinate newer initiatives such as the *Sampoorna Suraksha Strategy (SSS)* and other integrated service models, adapted to local epidemiological contexts **(Flowchart 5)**
Developing integrated communication strategies	Recognizing the shared behavioral and structural determinants of HIV and STIs, NACP promotes unified communication campaigns. These will cover awareness, risk reduction, testing, and treatment, and will be tailored by age, gender, and risk profile
Scaling up dual testing at HCTS centers	Rapid diagnostic test kits for *simultaneous detection of HIV and syphilis* will be expanded across service delivery points. These efforts will include structured algorithms for confirmatory testing, case management, and follow-up. Syphilis screening through *RPR testing* will be targeted at populations and locations with high prevalence

Continued

Continued

Goal 4: Promote universal access to quality STI/RTI services to at-risk and vulnerable populations.

Promoting active case finding	To detect STIs early, the program will intensify outreach using *social network-based testing, index case tracing*, and proactive risk screening in key populations
Collaborating with NHM on service provision and reporting	NACP will work closely with the National Health Mission to scale up STI prevention and management services across all levels of the health system. Emphasis will be placed on integrating diagnostics and linking clients to quality-assured care pathways **(Fig. 8)**
Engaging the private sector	Private healthcare providers, including those in the unorganized sector, will be brought into the national response through capacity building, standardized protocols, and reporting frameworks aligned with national guidelines
Regularizing the update of the STI/RTI management guidelines periodically	Advances in diagnostics—especially point-of-care multiplex tests for HIV, STIs, and Hepatitis—will inform the transition from syndromic to etiological treatment models **(Table 5)**. Emerging service delivery options such as telemedicine and self-care strategies are being piloted for broader implementation
Enhancing laboratory capacity	The existing three-tier STI laboratory network **(Fig. 9)** will be reviewed, restructured, and strengthened. Focus areas include diagnostic upgrades, antimicrobial resistance surveillance, and informed updates to national treatment policies
Strengthening supply chain systems	IT-enabled systems will be implemented to track supply and usage of STI diagnostic and treatment commodities, ensuring availability and reducing stock-outs across service delivery sites

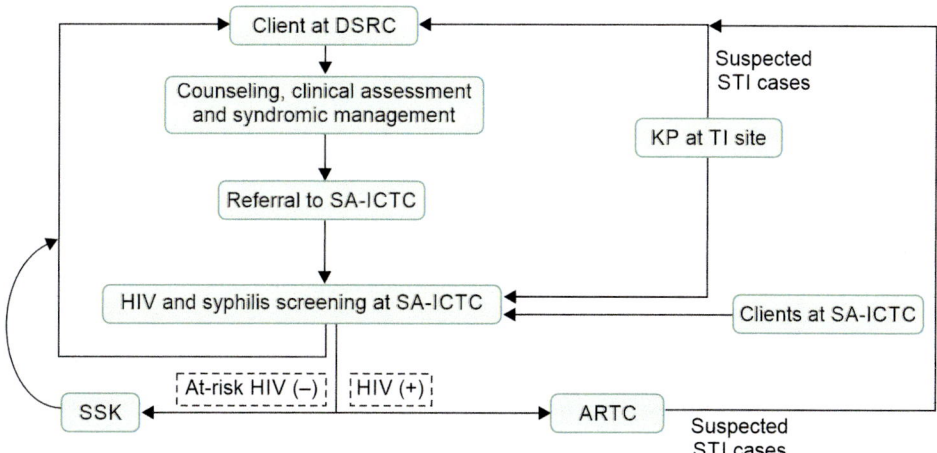

Note: There are in-referrals to DSRCs from other departments (including OBGY and DVD) of District Hospital/Medical Colleges.
FLOWCHART 5: Service delivery framework at designated STI/RTI clinics (DSRC).

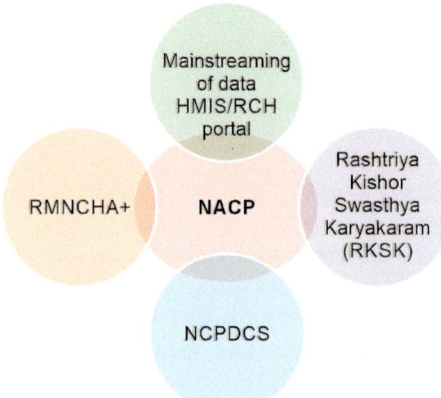

- Mainstreaming of HIV testing data reported through NHM portal, i.e., health management information system (HMIS) and reproductive and child health (RCH) portal
- Screening and management of STI/RTI services among adolescents through RKSK
- Screening and management of cervical cancer among WLHIV and FSWs through NCPDCS
- Case reporting system for syphilis among pregnant women and exposed children

FIG. 8: Collaboration with National Health Mission (NHM).

TABLE 5: Color-coded kits under NACP.

Kit	Composition	Targeted syndrome
Kit 1 (gray)	Tablet azithromycin 1,000 mg and cefixime 8,000 mg single-dose tablet	• Urethral discharge syndrome • Vaginal discharge syndrome (for cervicitis) • Painful scrotal swelling • Presumptive treatment (PT)
Kit 2 (green)	Tablet secnidazole 2,000 mg and tablet fluconazole 150 mg single dose	Vaginal discharge syndrome (for vaginitis)
Kit 3 (white)	• Injection benzathine penicillin G 2.4 MU • Azithromycin 1,000 mg single dose and tablet • Disposable syringe 10 mL with 21-gauge needle and sterile water 10 mL	Genital ulcer disease syndrome (for syphilis and chancroid)
Kit 4 (blue)	Tablet doxycycline 100 mg (28 capsules as twice/day dose for 14 days) and tablet azithromycin 1 g single dose	Genital ulcer disease syndrome (for syphilis and chancroid when unavailability or history of allergy to BPG)
Kit 5 (red)	Tablet acyclovir 400 mg (21 tablets as three times/day dose for 7 days)	Genital ulcer disease syndrome (for herpetic ulcers)
Kit 6 (yellow)	Tablet cefixime 800 mg single dose and tablet metronidazole 400 mg (28 tablets as twice/day dose for 14 days) and capsule doxycycline 100 mg (28 capsules as twice/day dose for 14 days)	Lower abdomen pain PID
Kit 7 (black)	Tablet doxycycline 100 mg (42 capsules as twice/day dose for 21 days)	• Inguinal bubo under genital ulcer disease syndrome • LGV proctitis under anorectal discharge syndrome
Kit 8 (brown)	Tablet cefixime 800 mg STAT dose and tablet doxycycline 100 mg (14 capsules as twice/day dose for 7 days)	Anorectal discharge syndrome

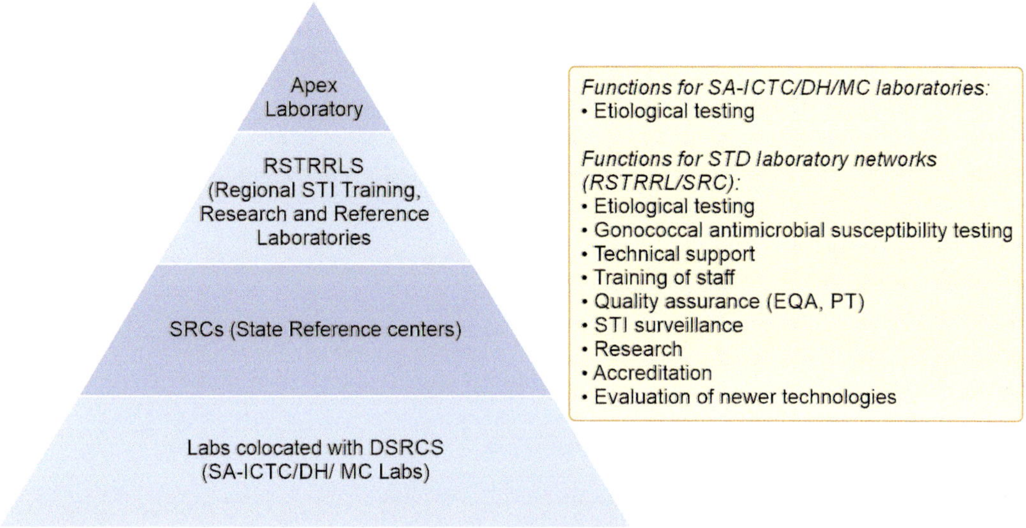

CHAPTER 8: Sexually Transmitted Infection Control Programs

Apex Laboratory

RSTRRLS (Regional STI Training, Research and Reference Laboratories)

SRCs (State Reference centers)

Labs colocated with DSRCS (SA-ICTC/DH/ MC Labs)

Functions for SA-ICTC/DH/MC laboratories:
- Etiological testing

Functions for STD laboratory networks (RSTRRL/SRC):
- Etiological testing
- Gonococcal antimicrobial susceptibility testing
- Technical support
- Training of staff
- Quality assurance (EQA, PT)
- STI surveillance
- Research
- Accreditation
- Evaluation of newer technologies

FIG. 9: STI laboratory network.

Goal 5: Eliminate HIV/AIDS-related stigma and discrimination.	
Institutionalizing community engagement	Community system strengthening (CSS) is being embedded into the program to ensure active participation of key populations (KPs) and PLHIV. These systems will support the design, delivery, and monitoring of services through grassroots-level leadership and feedback mechanisms **(Flowchart 6 and Boxes 3 and 4)**
Operationalizing legal provisions under the HIV Act, 2017	Efforts are underway to accelerate the notification of state-specific rules under the HIV and AIDS (Prevention and Control) Act, 2017. Each state will appoint an *ombudsman* and *complaints officers* at institutions to handle grievances related to discrimination and ensure enforcement of the Act
Stakeholder sensitization	Targeted capacity-building programs will be rolled out for key institutions—including workplaces, schools, and healthcare facilities—to raise awareness, reduce prejudice, and promote nondiscriminatory service delivery. These programs will educate stakeholders on legal provisions and build their ability to respond effectively
Strategic communication campaigns	Mass media, mid-media, and interpersonal communication approaches will be integrated into stigma-reduction campaigns **(Table 6)**. These campaigns will address misconceptions, promote empathy, and support behavior change. All communication efforts will include measurable indicators for tracking their effectiveness
Improving strategic information systems	New data collection tools will be introduced to assess stigma and discrimination across four key settings: Healthcare, community, workplace, and educational institutions. This evidence will guide targeted interventions and allow for regular impact evaluation
Promoting social protection schemes	Social welfare initiatives launched by state governments will be scaled up and aligned with the national HIV response. These schemes improve access to services and empower PLHIV and vulnerable populations by addressing barriers related to social exclusion, poverty, and marginalization

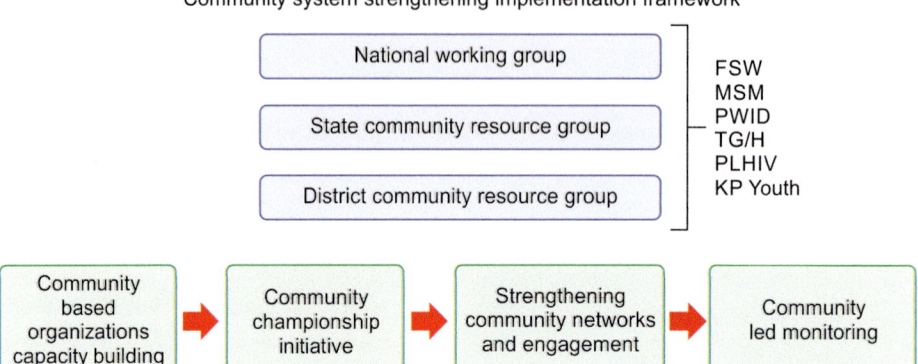

FLOWCHART 6: Implementation framework of community system strengthening.

BOX 3: Key aspects of community-led monitoring.
- CLM will play a central role in ensuring that program design and implementation reflect the needs of the community
- It involves routine feedback from people living with HIV (PLHIV) and key populations on the quality of services, challenges faced, and suggestions for improvement, especially around stigma, access, and retention in care

---

BOX 4: Key aspects of community champions.
- Influential individuals from within key population groups will be identified and trained as community champions
- These individuals will serve as advocates, educators, and mobilizers within their networks, helping to reduce stigma, encourage service uptake, and build community resilience

---

TABLE 6: Key aspects of information, education, and communication.

Information, education, and communication (IEC)	
Objectives of IEC: • Behavior change • Demand generation • Reduction of stigma and discrimination *A multimedia approach:* • Mass media (TV, radio, etc.) • Mid media (posters and special events) • Interpersonal communication (IPC) • SBCC	*Flagship initiatives:* • National Toll-free AIDS Helpline (1097) • Red Ribbon Express campaigns • Digital media outreach (social media, mobile apps) • Community events and school-based activities • Resource hubs and repositories for knowledge sharing

CONCLUSION

- India has the second largest estimated number of PLHIV (24 lakhs) in the world of which 40% are in Maharashtra, Andhra Pradesh, and Karnataka.
- Injecting drug users have the highest prevalence of HIV (9%).
- NACO has adopted 95-95-95 targets set by UNAIDS "to end HIV/AIDS as a Public Health threat by 2030".
- Quality standardized sexual and reproductive health services provided at district, subdistrict, and medical college level, through designated STI/RTI clinics (DSRC) or "Suraksha Clinics".
- NACP Phase V will focus on newer initiatives such as Sampoorna Suraksha Strategy to cover "at-risk" HIV negative but non-TI population through a cyclical and comprehensive package of services.
- NACP phase-V focuses on STI/RTI through the inclusion of Goal 3 and 4.
- Laboratory support for STI/RTI has been strengthened through a network of 10 regional STI laboratories and 45 state reference centers.

REFERENCES

1. National AIDS Control Organization. Strategy Document: National AIDS and STD Control Programme Phase-V (2021-26). New Delhi: NACO, Ministry of Health and Family Welfare, Government of India; 2022.
2. National Technical Guidelines on Sexually Transmitted Infections and Reproductive Tract Infections. (2024). National AIDS Control Organization, Ministry of Health and Family Welfare, Government of India.
3. Elimination of Vertical Transmission of HIV & Syphilis. Guidelines. National AIDS & STD Control Programme. Ministry of Health & Family Welfare, India; 2023.

CHAPTER 9

Recent Advances in Management of Sexually Transmitted Diseases

Yashpal Manchanda, Sudip Das

INTRODUCTION

Sexually transmitted infections (STIs) have recently witnessed an upward trend especially after the COVID-19 pandemic.[1,2] They have now become the second most common group of infections after the respiratory infections. As per World Health Organization (WHO), >1 million cases of STIs are being diagnosed every single day globally.[3] Thus, there is an urgent requirement to contain the spread of these infections. Implementation of recent advances made in the diagnosis, treatment, and prevention of these conditions forms an effective tool to achieve the objective. Equally important is the dissemination of information interlaced with interventions, along with the emphasis on measures aimed at building a healthier society. As it has been done with tobacco, alcohol, diet, and lifestyle diseases.[4] In this chapter, we will deal with the recent advances made in diagnosis, management, and prevention of the four major STIs [gonorrhea, syphilis, chlamydia, and human immunodeficiency virus (HIV)] including new rapid diagnostic tests, novel vaccines, preexposure prophylaxis (prep) beyond HIV, and long-acting (LA) antiviral agents.

Also, COVID-19 pandemic proved to be a blessing in disguise and lead to an exponential rise in number of patients utilizing telemedicine services, leading to remarkable improvement in accessibility of diagnostic tests as well as on line drug prescription of STIs.[5-7] Thereby, allowing patients to consult healthcare providers and receive drug prescriptions remotely.

SYPHILIS

Quick and highly sensitive diagnostic tests are key to STI management and transmission interruption. In recent times, especially because of COVID-19, there has been a rapid development in newer STI testing approaches.[8] Mostly, because of pandemic associated problems with traditional STI testing, e.g., supply chain disruptions, administrative movement restrictions, fear of catching the deadly virus infection, closed STD clinics, or an overwhelmed laboratory staff. Resultant to which, new web-based companies offering STI test and remote laboratories have cropped up.[9] Huge success of self-testing COVID kit has paved the way for similar STI testing kit. Recently self-testing HIV kit was introduced in the market.[10] Because of the current nonavailability of similar tests for other STIs, there has been an emergence of home specimen self-collection models with send-off to testing laboratory. Testing for syphilis is more challenging to include in telehealth models.[11] Serologic tests require blood collection. A point-of-care dual testing (POCT) method for simultaneous detection of HIV and syphilis developed recently, is being used in multiple countries, e.g., The Syphilis Health Check Treponemal Antibody test (SHC, Trinity Biotech) and DPP® HIV-Syphilis System by Chembio Diagnostic Systems Inc, which is a rapid HIV/syphilis test.[12] Both, SHC and DPP are treponemal antibody screening tests and need to be followed up with a laboratory-based nontreponemal test, if found to be positive. Both these tests do not need phlebotomy, and can be done on a drop of blood from finger prick. These tests can be read within 15 minutes by without any additional device for SHC, or with the help of a small reader in case of DPP. They have the potential to bring rapid testing closer to people's homes and provide greater access, speed, and convenience.[13]

Human Immunodeficiency Virus

Rapid HIV diagnostic tests have been available for more than a decade now, resulting in increased accessibility during screening campaigns and for other outreach programs. However, the patient had to still visit a healthcare facility. Most of the high-risk cases are already marginalized in the society, and they avoided visiting healthcare facility for the fear of being victimized. Thus, the testing services delivery to the target population required innovation. Recently, with the commercial availability of US Food and Drug Administration (FDA) approved rapid oral HIV diagnostic kits at retail stores across the United States.[10] A new opportunity of expanding the HIV screening and monitoring services has become available. OraQuick In-Home HIV testing kit from OraSure Technologies, Inc (Bethlehem, PA) was first such test to get US FDA approval. It can detect antibodies against both HIV 1 and 2 from just an oral swab, and gives the result within 20 minutes, providing a confidential in-home testing option.

In the beginning of 21st century, important breakthrough in prevention of HIV occurred. It was shown that administering antiretroviral (ARV) drugs to uninfected individuals engaged in high-risk practices significantly reduced their chances of acquiring HIV.[14] Thus, prEP was promoted among MSM and CSWs. As a result, significant reduction in the incidence of newer HIV infection has been witnessed in last one decade. The rate has halved to 1.5 million/year in 2021, from 3 million/year in 2000. The older medications were required to be taken orally daily and there were issues with compliance. But, with the recent introduction of potent LA ARVs in combination with the advances in controlled release technologies has enabled LA ARV drug delivery systems (DDS) capable of providing extended dosing intervals.[15-17] And thus, have overcome the challenge of suboptimal drug adherence with daily oral dosing. The LA injectable (LAI) ARV therapy, as well as its use for prEP, has further given renewed hope for the possibility of ending the HIV epidemic. As of 2021, the use of LAI in prEP has been approved by US FDA. LAI antiretroviral therapy (ART) includes administration of a combination of cabotegravir and rilpivirine every 8 weeks. Similarly, the dapivirine vaginal ring (DVR) has recently become an additional LA preventative option.[18] It is a flexible silicone vaginal ring that releases dapivirine, a non-nucleoside reverse transcriptase inhibitor (NNRTI) and provides protection against acquiring HIV for up to 1 month. One such method for the development of potent LA ARV, being explored is by developing modified prodrug for the existing ARVs, which enables them to be packed in a capsule, ready to be used in LA DDS. Various approaches are being tried for prodrug modification. One such successful approach is "ProTide approach", it is used for intracellular delivery of nucleotide analogs. Wherein, the active phosphate group of the ARV is masked with an amino acid ester and an aryl moiety. The prodrug is then subsequently encapsulated into poloxamer nanocrystals to prolong its half-life, and for efficient intracellular delivery.[19,20] It has been used to increase the plasma stability as well as to mask the toxicity of tenofovir (TFV), by developing TAF prodrug. Similarly, it has also been used for lamivudine (3TC) and emtricitabine (FTC). And, is also being evaluated for other newer ARVs which are still under various developmental stages. One such example of a recently patented drug is GS-9131 (rovafovir etalafenamide) for the nucleoside analog GS-9148. Other techniques for prodrug modification are lipophilic fatty acid ester prodrug, drug polymer conjugates.

On the advanced controlled release technology front, subcutaneous and/or subdermal implants have been developed that provide controlled drug release for prolonged periods for up to 1 year. Several of these implants containing potent ARV drugs are under various stages of development. They provide an added advantage of removal in case of drug reaction or sensitivity. Biodegradable implants have the advantage that they do not need to be removed, after the drug has finished. One such advancement in this category is the "in situ forming implants (ISFI)".[21] These are basically ARV in polymeric solution form, which when injected into the body solidify, and release the drug slowly over longer periods up to 9 months to 1 year.

Finally, transdermal LA patches, oral LA ARV formulations are some of other avenues under developmental stages and being tried in animals. Which shall soon be available for human use, and are expected to simplify the ARV administration further by avoiding hospital visit for insertion or removal of implant, or even contact with healthcare worker (HCW) for injections.

Although advances made in the ART have led to significant suppression of HIV replication as well as reduction in incidence of new cases. However, severe adverse reaction and inability of these agents to target integrated proviral genome are the two important issues that still remain to be addressed.[19] These unmet needs in fight against HIV has lead the researchers to a completely new field of gene-based therapies. Clustered Regularly Interspaced Short Palindromic Repeats (CRISPR), is one such gene editing tool being extensively studied by many scientists. And, CRISPR-associated protein-9 nuclease (Cas9) has proved to be an effective genome editing tool in the last decade.[22] And, has been used to target the integrated proviral HIV-1 genome, both in in vitro as well as in vivo studies including nonhuman primates. This has also been tested in latent HIV-1 infection, by modulating the proviral transcription using Cas9 mutant developed specifically for this purpose. Thus, in near future CRISPR seems to hold lot of promise as a primary genome editing tool for eradicating HIV-1 infection.

Gonorrhea

It is very concerning to note that *Neisseria gonorrhoeae* (NG) has become resistant to almost all antimicrobial agents previously recommended in the guidelines for the treatment of gonorrhea including macrolide, fluoroquinolones, and even extended spectrum cephalosporins.[23] After having noticed this alarming trend, WHO published guidelines to mitigate the emergence and spread of antimicrobial resistance (AMR) in NG. Advocating the use of nucleic acid amplification tests at the point-of-care (POC), instead of conventional culture methods for quicker detection of AMR mechanism or determinants to predict NG AMR, and earlier initiation of personalized treatment for NG.[24,25] There are ongoing efforts to develop microfluidic and nanotechnology-based approaches to find low technology and even equipment-free assays, that could be offered at POC even in remotest of areas. Two new drugs that have evolved for ceftriaxone-resistant gonorrhoea are zoliflodacin (FDA approved) and gepotidacin with 93% cure rate. In future, whole genome sequencing (WGS)-based methods are likely to replace NAAT-based testing for NG AMR prediction, offering a 360° genetic view of the strains and samples. In fact, WGS has a distinct advantage of detecting all known and not previously discovered AMR determinants at the same time.[26]

Recent STI treatment guidelines have recommended the use of single dose combination of injection ceftriaxone 250 mg intramuscularly and azithromycin 1 g orally as first-line treatment for uncomplicated gonorrhea.[27] Alternatively, single dose combination of cefixime 400 mg and azithromycin 1 g can also be given, which works out well in field conditions.

Regarding the development of effective gonococcal vaccine, the progress made so far has been very slow.[28] Which is largely due to the fact that NG is characterized by very high degree of antigenic variations. Thus, making it difficult to find a suitable immunogenicity to develop an effective vaccine.[29] However, recently researchers have identified that TonB-dependent transporters (TdTs) produced by NG play an important role in helping the organism to survive in the nutrient depleted conditions encountered in the human host. Also, these TdTs are generally well conserved across the NG species, and do not undergo phase variations. Which make them suitable targets for vaccine development. Currently, research is ongoing to develop antisera against the hybrid TbpA antigens. Another NG antigen, which has generated interest as a candidate for vaccine development is gonococcal lipooligosaccharide (LOS). Its epitomes have been researched for possible use in vaccine development. Recently, it has been shown that the 2C7 epitope of NG LOS is mostly conserved amongst all strains, and stays immunogenic during the course of natural infection. And, thus has attracted attention as a potential vaccine target.[30,31] In a recent study a peptide mimic of this epitome, also called as "Mimitome", when given along with Th1 stimulating adjuvant showed to generate immunoglobulin G (IgG) antibodies bactericidal to the NG in an experimentally infected mice.[32]

CHLAMYDIA

Chlamydia trachomatis (CT) is an obligate intracellular pathogen with a biphasic developmental cycle consisting of infectious elementary body (EB) and replicative reticulate body (RB), these characteristics have long acted as the main hurdles in developing tools for its genetic manipulaton.[33] However, in the past decade significant progress has been made in this domain, including chemical mutagenesis, group II intron-based targeted gene knockout, fluorescence-reported allelic exchange mutagenesis (FRAEM), CRISPR interference (CRISPRi), and most recently transposon mutagenesis.

The first portable, CLIA-waived test termed "Sexual Health Test" (Visby MedicalTM) for chlamydia, gonorrhea, and *Trichomonas vaginalis* detection was cleared in August 2021.[34] It is a 30-minute PCR test performed on a disposable, single use, handheld device. As of now, it is approved for self-collected vaginal swabs in a healthcare setting.

Currently, vaccines for CT and NG are still in development phase or at the most being tested in clinical trials.[35]

HUMAN PAPILLOMAVIRUS

Human papillomavirus (HPV)-related vaccines have been developed and deployed in recent times, both as an immunotherapeutic agent for genital warts and cervical cancer as well as in prophylaxis against cervical cancer.[36] At least three HPV vaccines are licensed in the United States: Cervarix, a

2-valent vaccine (2vHPV) that targets HPV types 16 and 18; Gardasil, a 4-valent vaccine (4vHPV) that targets HPV types 6, 11, 16, and 18; and, the most recent Gardasil 9, a 9-valent vaccine (9vHPV) that targets HPV types 6, 11, 16, 18, 31, 33, 45, 52, and 58. National guidelines for HPV vaccination vary from country to country depending upon the availability and prevailing local conditions. However, Advisory Committee on Immunization Practices (ACIP) in US recommends to vaccinate all adolescents at the age of 11-12 years. For those, who missed the vaccine at this age, a Catch-up vaccination is recommended for older adolescents and young adults through age 26 years. The doses of vaccine vary depending upon the age. A two-dose vaccine schedule given at 0 and 6-12-month intervals is recommended for the cases < 15 years of age. But, in cases with immunosuppression, it is recommended to give three doses at 0, 1-2, and then at 6-12 months, regardless of age of the patient. Importantly, all the doses need to be administered within 1 year.[37]

TRICHOMONAS VAGINALIS

Recently, Helicase-dependent amplification technique-based molecular diagnostic tests have become available, which can be used for rapid detection of *T. vaginalis* even in asymptomatic women, using either vaginal or even urine specimens, thereby allowing at POC diagnosis and management.[38] These tests work on the principle of unique primer-based amplification of *T. vaginalis*-specific target sequence. And, there are numerous such US FDA approved tests available commercially now, at least in the developed countries. With very high sensitivity rates of over and above 98% for vaginal specimens, and >92% for urine, in comparison to standard nucleic acid amplification tests (NAAT). AmpliVue® is one such test, which does not require large machines to analyze the results, and is done with the help of small hand held cartridge. There is another very rapid *T. vaginalis* antigen detecting diagnostic test based on immunochromatographic assay, available as OSOM®, which is again very easy and gives results in 10-15 minutes, and is well suited for STI screening campaigns carried out in remote areas under field conditions in resource poor countries. It is also a validated tool for the diagnosis of *T. vaginalis* in women, and has a sensitivity of 83-92% and specificity of 99% for clinician-obtained vaginal specimens.[39]

Although, as per Centers for Disease Control and Prevention (CDC) STIs treatment guidelines published in 2015. The first-line treatment of *T. vaginalis* in HIV-negative patients remains tablet metronidazole (MTZ) 2 g stat dose given orally.[40] Alternatively, MTZ given in dose of 500 mg twice daily orally for 7 days, has been recommended, in HIV positive patients. But, recent meta-analysis of treatment trials of trichomonas infection showed that women receiving 500 mg twice daily MTZ regimen were 50% more likely to be negative for infection at test of cure (TOC), in comparison to those given 2 g stat dose therapy.[41] Similar results were also witnessed in randomized controlled trials (RCTs) comparing HIV positive with HIV-negative women having *T. Vaginalis* infection. Thus, current consensus is to treat all patients with 7-day regimen.[42] Moreover, recent literature review did not find any increased risk of teratogenicity with the use of MTZ during pregnancy (Class B drug).

In case of persistent or recurrent infection due to treatment failure, and if the possibility of reinfection has been excluded. These patients can still be successfully treated with little longer courses or additional doses of MTZ or tinidazole (TIN). In case of treatment failure with 7-day regimen of high-dose oral MTZ or TIN, two additional treatment regimens that can be successfully used are—high-dose oral TIN 2-3 g daily plus intravaginal TIN 500 mg twice daily for 14 days, or high-dose oral TIN plus intravaginal paromomycin cream for 14 days.[43] The rise of STIs have led to use of doxycycline in pre- and postexposure.[44]

CONCLUSION

Overall, with the rates of chlamydia, gonorrhea, and syphilis continue to surge with each passing year, compounded by the growing incidence of antibiotic resistance even to newer drugs. There is an urgent need to address the issue of sexually transmitted infections in a multi pronged fashion, involving all the stake holders at every level. And, dissemination of knowledge amongst the healthcare workers about the recent advancements being made in the field of sexually transmitted infections constitutes one of the most important component of the strategy. Only through such repeated concerted efforts, the barriers to resources and education can be broken down. And, hopefully with this, knowledge of health sexual encounters and resources for treatment, the transmission rates of the sexually transmitted infections should be brought under control, and should in fact start falling in near future.

REFERENCES

1. Williamson DA, Chen MY. Emerging and reemerging sexually transmitted infections. N Eng J Med. 2020;382:2023-32.
2. Soriano V, Blasco-Fontecilla H, Gallego L, Fernández-Montero JV, Mendoza C, Barreiro P. Rebound in sexually transmitted infections after the COVID-19 pandemic. AIDS Rev. 2023;26(3):127-35.
3. WHO. (2022). WHO report on Sexually Transmitted Infections (STI's). [online] Available from: https://www.who.int/news-room/fact-sheets/details/sexually-transmitted-infections-(stis) [Last accessed June, 2025].
4. Akter S, Islam MR, Rahman MM, Rouyard T, Nsashiyi RS, Hossain F, et al. Evaluation of Population-Level Tobacco Control Interventions and Health Outcomes: A Systematic Review and Meta-Analysis. JAMA Netw Open. 2023;6(7):e2322341.
5. Ogunbodede OT, Zablotska-Manos I, Lewis DA. Potential and demonstrated impacts of the COVID-19 pandemic on sexually transmissible infections. Curr Opin Infect Dis. 2021;34(1):56-61.
6. Valentine JA, Mena L, Millett G. Telehealth Services: Implications for Enhancing Sexually Transmitted Infection Prevention. Sex Transm Dis. 2022;49(1S Suppl 2):S36-S40.
7. Kersh EN, Shukla M, Raphael BH, Habel M, Park I. At-Home Specimen Self-Collection and Self-Testing for Sexually Transmitted Infection Screening Demand Accelerated by the COVID-19 Pandemic: a Review of Laboratory Implementation Issues. J Clin Microbiol. 2021;59(11):e0264620.
8. Boum Y, Eyangoh S, Okomo MC. Beyond COVID-19-will self-sampling and testing become the norm? Lancet Infect Dis. 2021;21(9):1194-5.
9. Kersh EN. Advances in STI Testing at Home and in Non-Clinical Settings Close to the Home. Sex Transm Dis. 2022;49(11):S12-4.
10. Hecht J, Sanchez T, Sullivan PS, DiNenno EA, Cramer N, Delaney KP. Increasing Access to HIV Testing Through Direct-to-Consumer HIV Self-Test Distribution- United States, March 31, 2020-March 30, 2021. MMWR Morb Mortal Wkly Rep. 2021;70(38):1322-5.
11. Bristow CC, Klausner JD, Tran A. Clinical test performance of a rapid point-of-care syphilis treponemal antibody test: A systematic review and meta-analysis. Clin Infect Dis. 2020; 71(Suppl 1):S52-7.
12. T Naidu P, Tsang RS. Canadian Public Health Laboratory Network guidelines for the use of point-of-care tests for *Treponema pallidum* in Canada. J Assoc Med Microbiol Infect Dis Can. 2022;7(2):85-96.
13. Riegler AN, Larsen N, Amerson-Brown MH. Point-of-care testing for sexually transmitted infections. Clin Lab Med. 2023;43(2):189-207.
14. Tuddenham S, Hamill MM, Ghanem KG. Diagnosis and Treatment of Sexually Transmitted Infections: A Review. JAMA. 2022;327(2):161-72.
15. Thoueille P, Choong E, Cavassini M, Buclin T, Decosterd LA. Long-acting antiretrovirals: a new & era for the management and prevention

of HIV infection. J Antimicrob Chemother. 2022;77(2):290-302.
16. Swindells S, Lutz T, van Zyl L, Porteiro N, Stoll M, Mitha E, et al. Long-acting cabotegravir+ rilpivirine for HIV-1 treatment: ATLAS week 96 results. AIDS. 2022;36:185-94.
17. Goebel MC, Guajardo E, Giordano TP, Patel SM. The New Era of Long-Acting Antiretroviral Therapy: When and Why to Make the Switch. Curr HIV/AIDS Rep. 2023;20(5):271-85.
18. Krovi SA, Johnson LM, Luecke E, Achilles SL, van der Straten A. Advances in long-acting injectables, implants, and vaginal rings for contraception and HIV prevention. Adv Drug Deliv Rev. 2021;176:113849.
19. Landovitz RJ, Kofron R, McCauley M. The promise and pitfalls of long acting injectable agents for HIV prevention. Curr Opin HIV AIDS. 2016;11:122-8.
20. Scarsi KK, Swindells S. The promise of improved adherence with long-acting antiretroviral therapy: what are the data? J Int Assoc Provid AIDS Care. 2021;20:23259582211009012.
21. Coulter SM, Pentlavalli S, An Y, Vora LK, Cross ER, Moore JV, et al. In Situ Forming, Enzyme-Responsive Peptoid-Peptide Hydrogels: An Advanced Long-Acting Injectable Drug Delivery System. J Am Chem Soc. 2024;146(31):21401-16.
22. Bhowmik R, Chaubey B. CRISPR/Cas9: a tool to eradicate HIV-1. AIDS Res Ther. 2022;19(1):58.
23. Unemo M, Shafer WM. Antimicrobial resistance in *Neisseria gonorrhoeae* in the 21st century: past, evolution, and future. Clin Microbiol Rev. 2014;27(3):587-613
24. World Health Organization. Global action plan to control the spread and impact of antimicrobial resistance in *Neisseria gonorrhoeae*. Geneva (Switzerland): World Health Organization; 2012.
25. World Health Organization. WHO guidelines for the treatment of *Neisseria gonorrhoeae*. Geneva (Switzerland): World Health Organization; 2016.
26. Donà V, Low N, Golparian D, Unemo M. Recent advances in the development and use of molecular tests to predict antimicrobial resistance in *Neisseria gonorrhoeae*. Expert Rev Mol Diagn. 2017;17(9):845-59.
27. Garrett NJ, Osman F, Maharaj B, Naicker N, Gibbs A, Norman E, et al. Beyond syndromic management: Opportunities for diagnosis-based treatment of sexually transmitted infections. in low- and middle-income countries. PLoS One. 2018;13(4):e0196209.
28. Maurakis SA, Cornelissen CN. Recent Progress Towards a Gonococcal Vaccine. Front Cell Infect Microbiol. 2022;12:881392.
29. Maurakis S, Keller K, Maxwell CN, Pereira K, Chazin WJ, Criss AK, et al. The Novel Interaction Between *Neisseria Gonorrhoeae* Tdfj and Human S100A7 Allows Gonococci to Subvert Host Zinc Restriction. PloS Pathog. 2019;15:e1007937.
30. Gulati S, Shaughnessy J, Ram S, Rice PA. Targeting Lipooligosaccharide (LOS) for a Gonococcal Vaccine. Front Immunol. 2019;10:321.
31. Ram S, Gulati S, Lewis L A, Chakraborti S, Zheng B, Deoliveira RB, et al. A Novel Sialylation Site on *Neisseria Gonorrhoeae* Lipooligosaccharide Links Heptose II Lactose Expression With Pathogenicity. Infect Immun. 2018;86:e00285-18.
32. Waltmann A, Chen JS, Duncan JA. Promising developments in gonococcal vaccines. Curr Opin Infect Dis. 2024;37(1):63-9.
33. Chavda VP, Pandya A, Kypreos E, Patravale V, Apostolopoulos V. *Chlamydia trachomatis*: quest for an eye-opening vaccine breakthrough. Expert Rev Vaccines. 2022;21(6):771-81.
34. Lockhart A, Psioda M, Ting J, Campbell S, Mugo N, Kwatampora J, et al. Prospective Evaluation of Cervicovaginal Self- and Cervical Physician Collection for the Detection of *Chlamydia trachomatis, Neisseria gonorrhoeae, Trichomonas vaginalis,* and *Mycoplasma genitalium* Infections. Sex Transm Dis. 2018;45(7):488-93.
35. Poston TB. Advances in vaccine development for *Chlamydia trachomatis*. Pathog Dis. 2024;82:ftae017.
36. Nilyanimit P, Vichaiwattana P, Aeemchinda R, Bhunyakitikorn W, Thantithaveewat T, Seetho S, et al. Effectiveness of HPV vaccine as part of national immunization program for preventing HPV infection in Thai schoolgirls after seven years post-vaccination. Hum Vaccin Immunother. 2024;20(1):2392330.
37. Markowitz LE, Naleway AL, Klein NP, Lewis RM, Crane B, Querec TD, et al. Human Papillomavirus Vaccine Effectiveness Against HPV Infection: Evaluation of One, Two, and Three Doses. J Infect Dis. 2020;221(6):910-8.
38. Gaydos CA, Schwebke J, Dombrowski J, Marrazzo J, Coleman J, Silver B, et al. Clinical performance of the Solana® Point-of-Care Trichomonas Assay from clinician-collected vaginal swabs and urine specimens from symptomatic and asymptomatic women. Expert Rev Mol Diagn. 2017;17(3):303-6.
39. Schwebke JR, Gaydos CA, Davis T, Marrazzo J, Furgerson D, Taylor SN, et al. Clinical Evaluation of the Cepheid Xpert TV Assay for Detection of Trichomonas vaginalis with Prospectively Collected Specimens from Men and Women. J Clin Microbiol. 2018;56(2):pii:64.e01091-17.

40. Workowski KA, Bachmann LH, Chan PA, Johnston CM, Muzny CA, Park I, et al. Sexually Transmitted Infections Treatment Guidelines, 2021. MMWR Recomm Rep. 2021;70(4):1-187.
41. Howe K, Kissinger PJ. Single-Dose Compared With Multidose Metronidazole for the Treatment of Trichomoniasis in Women: A Meta-Analysis. Sex Transm Dis. 2017;44(1):29-34.
42. Kissinger P, Muzny CA, Mena LA, Lillis RA, Schwebke JR, Beauchamps L, et al. Single-dose versus 7-day-dose metronidazole for the treatment of trichomoniasis in women: an open-label, randomized controlled trial. Lancet Infect Dis. 2018;18(11):1251-9.
43. Muzny CA, Van Gerwen OT, Kissinger P. Updates in trichomonas treatment including persistent infection and 5-nitroimidazole hypersensitivity. Curr Opin Infect Dis. 2020;33(1):73-7.
44. Stratman S, Zampella JG. Review of doxycycline prophylaxis of sexually transmitted infections. J Eur Acad Dermatol Venereol. 2025;39:1091-8.

Index

Page numbers followed by *b* refer to box, *f* refer to figure, *fc* refer to flowchart, and *t* refer to table.

A

Acneiform eruptions 35
Acquired immunodeficiency syndrome 4, 66*t*
    prevention and control act 4, 66, 67
    related mortalities 72
Activator protein-1 28
Acyclovir 5, 11, 12, 78
Adenovirus 21
    Candida species 18
Adolescent immunization programs 58
Advisory Committee on Immunization
        Practices 86
Allelic exchange mutagenesis 85
Amine test, positive 14
Amino acid 83
Amsel's clinical criteria 16
Anaerobic gram-negative bacilli 14
Anal fistulae 10
Anal intraepithelial neoplasia 41
Anal pruritus 19
Angular stomatitis 35
Anogenital fibrosis 10
Anogenital warts 24
Anorectal discharge syndrome 5
Antibiotic-resistant strains, emergence of 57
Antimicrobial resistance, spread of 84
Antiretroviral drugs, administering 83
Antiretroviral therapy 73, 83
Anxiety disorders 52
Arthralgias 36
Azithromycin 5, 23, 48, 85

B

Bacillary angiomatosis 43
    diagnosis of 44
Bacillus Calmette-Guérin 29
Bacteria 4
Bacterial infection, streptococcal 44
Bacterial vaginosis 3, 14, 16, 17*f*
    and pregnancy 16
    clue cells indicating 15*f*
Bacteroides 14
Bartholin's gland abscess 20
Bartonella henselae 43
Bartonella quintana 43
Behavior change 69
Behavioural surveillance survey 2
Benzathine penicillin 12
Benzoin, tincture of 29
Bisexual 47, 52
Bleomycin injection 29
Breastfeeding women 12
Bull head clap 20*f*
Buschke-Lowenstein tumor 27

C

Candida
    albicans 4, 14, 17
    antigen 29
    colonization 40
Candidiasis 3, 43
Carbon dioxide laser therapy 30
CD4+ cell count 35*t*, 35, 42
CD4+ lymphocytes 26
CD4+ Th cells 34
Cecolin 57
Cefixime 5, 23, 85
Cell
    culture 21
    infected 21*f*
    protein, segment of infected 61
Cellulitis 44
Cervarix 31, 56, 57
Cervical
    cancer 85
        ranks 55
    discharge 23*t*, 23
    mucosa 39
Cervicitis 18
Cervix, strawberry appearance of 22*f*
Chancroid 3, 9, 39
Child sexual abuse 51
    signs of 51*b*

Chlamydia 1, 3, 21f, 55, 56, 82, 85
   rates of 87
   trachomatis 4, 8, 18, 21, 22f, 39, 59, 47, 48, 56, 85
Chlamydial protease 60
Chlamydial urethritis 21
   diagnosis of 21
Ciprofloxacin 11
   multidrug-resistant 48
Clindamycin 16
Clue cells 16
Coccidioidomycosis 43
Coliform bacteria 18
Colpitis macularis 16
Communication, key aspects of 80t
Community champions, key aspects of 80b
Community Health Center 6, 73
Community system strengthening, implementation framework of 80fc
Community-based integrated service models 69
Community-led monitoring 80b
Condyloma accuminata 24, 27
Conjunctivitis 22f
Counseling 5
COVID-19 pandemic 82
Cryotherapy 30
Cryptococcosis 35
Cyclophosphamide, low-dose 27

D

Dapivirine vaginal ring 83
Decentralized high-impact program management 68
Depression 51
Depressive symptoms, moderate-to-severe 52
Dermatophytosis 35
Dermoscopy 27
Disease
   burden and unmet need 55, 59, 61
   severe 42
Disseminated gonococcal infection 20f
Disseminated herpes zoster 42
Distal shaft, swelling of 20f
Döderlein's lactobacilli 14
Donovanosis 10, 13
Doxycycline 5, 11, 12
Drug
   delivery systems 83
   polymer conjugates 84
Dry skin 37

E

Ebola virus 48, 50
Ectocervicitis 18
Education, key aspects of 80t
Efficient intracellular delivery 84
Electrofulguration 30
Electrosurgery 30
Elephantiasis 10
Emtricitabine 84
Encephalitis 42
Endocervicitis 18
Entamoeba
   histolytica 48
   infection ranges 48
Enzyme-linked immunosorbent assay 20
Eosinophilic folliculitis 37
Epididymitis 20
Epitome 85
Erythema multiforme major 35
Erythematous papules 37f
Erythromycin 12
Esophageal candidiasis 43
Esophagitis 42
Evidence-based planning and monitoring 68

F

Famciclovir 11, 12
Femoral lymphadenopathy 10
Flagellated protozoa 21
Fluconazole 5
Fluoroquinolones 84
Fluorouracil 28
Fungal infections 42
Fungi 4

G

Gardasil 31, 56, 57, 86
Gay 47, 52
Genital chlamydia trachomatis 60
Genital discharge 3
Genital herpes 8, 55
   primary infection 12
   recurrent infection 12
   suppressive therapy 12
   treatment of 12t
Genital tract tissue 60
Genital ulcers 8, 35
   disease 3, 8, 40, 61
   syndrome 5
   swabs 10

Index

Genital vaccines 55
Genital warts 26f, 27, 41f
    pathogenesis of 25fc
    treatment of 28t, 29t
Gentamicin 11
Giemsa stain 21
Glans 9
Glycoprotein B2 61
Gonococcal lipooligosaccharide 85
Gonococcal urethritis 18, 19
    treatment of 21
Gonococcal vaccine 57
Gonococcus 56
Gonorrhea 1, 3, 55, 56, 82, 84
    current control measures for 57
    treatment of 84
Gram staining 18, 21
Guillain–Barré syndrome, increased risk of 50

H

Haemophilus
    ducreyi 8
    species 18
Harnessing technology and innovation 68
Headache 8
Healthcare
    setting 66
    worker 84
Heat-killed parasites, doses of 59
Hemorrhage, subconjunctival 52
Hepatitis
    A virus 49, 56
        transmitted sexually 49
    B virus 4, 56
    C virus 4, 48
Herpes simplex virus 1, 3, 4, 18, 21, 35, 41, 44, 56, 61
Herpes zoster 35
    chronic and recurrent 42
    persistent 42
Herpetic ulcers, chronic 41
Herpevac formulation 62
Histoplasma capsulatum 43
Histoplasmosis 43
Human immunodeficiency virus 1, 3, 4, 8, 16, 33, 38, 56, 66, 82, 83
    beneficiaries, care for 71
    care, support, and treatment services 73f
    cutaneous manifestations of 33
    disease, clinical features in 33
    eliminate vertical transmission of 74
    epidemic, global 2023 34f
    infections 69
    laboratory services 73f
    positive 41f
    prevention and control 66, 67
    prevention of parent-to-child transmission of 5
    scope of 66t
    syndrome, acute 36
    testing services 5
    transmission, risk of 65
Human papillomavirus 1, 4, 35, 55, 56, 85
    infection 40
    recombinant vaccine, bivalent 31
    vaccines 31t, 55, 57t

I

Ichthyosis 35
Idiopathic pruritus 35
Imiquimod 28
Immune
    enzyme assays 44
    system 34
Immunochromatographic assay 86
Immunofluorescence assays 44
Immunoglobulin G, detection of 44
Immunotherapy 29
In situ forming implants 84
Infection 56
    recurrent 86
Infectious elementary body 85
Inflammatory dermatoses 36
Information, education, and communication, key aspects of 80t
Inguinal lymphadenopathy 10
Inguinal swelling 3
Inmates postrelease 69
Integrated counseling and testing centres 5
Interferons alpha 29
Intra-amniotic infections 16
Intracellular diplococci 20f
Intravaginal paromomycin cream 87
Invasive meningococcal infection, clusters of 49
Isotretinoin 27

K

Kaposi's sarcoma 35, 44
Klebsiella granulomatis 10

L

Lactobacillus
  species 14
  strains 59
Lamivudine, used for 84
Laser therapy 30
Lentivirus 33
Leprosy 35
Lesbian 47, 52
Lifestyle diseases 82
Lipophilic fatty acid ester prodrug 84
Lymph nodes 10
Lymphadenopathy 40
Lymphogranuloma venereum 3, 5, 8, 10, 40, 48
  infection 48

M

Macrolide 84
Malaise 8, 36
Malodorous discharge 14
Measles, mumps, and rubella 29
Meningococcal B vaccine 57
Meningococcal serogroup B vaccine 57
Mental disorder, lifetime 52
Messenger ribonucleic acid-LNP vaccine, modified 62
Metastatic complications 20
Methicillin-resistant *Staphylococcus aureus* 48, 49
Metronidazole 16, 21, 59, 86
Migratory polyarthritis 20
Mimitome 85
Mission Sampark 66
Molluscum contagiosum 4, 35, 42, 42f, 35
Monkeypox 48, 50
  virus 4, 56
Mucocutaneous disorders 35
  prevalence of specific 35t
Myalgias 8, 36
Mycoplasma genitalium 18, 21, 39, 48, 49, 53

N

National AIDS and STD Control Programme 65f, 65, 67t
  collaborating agencies under 68f
  color-coded kits under 78t
  guiding principles of 67, 68b
  virtual interventions under 71t
National AIDS Control Organization 4, 4t, 71
National Health Mission 78f
Needle-syringe exchange program 69

Neisseria
  gonorrhoeae 18, 19, 39, 47, 56, 57
  meningitidis 18, 48, 49
Neonatal complications 56
Night sweats 36
Nongonococcal urethritis 18, 21
  infective causes 19f
Non-nucleoside reverse transcriptase inhibitor 83
Nontreponemal antibody testing 75f
Nontreponemal test, laboratory-based 83
Nuclear factor-kappa B 28
Nucleic acid amplification tests 10, 18, 20, 39, 86
Nucleoside, trivalent 62
Nucleoside-modified mRNA delivered 61
Nugent scoring 16

O

Odynophagia 43
One-stop centers 70b
  flow of services 71fc
  staff 71fc
Ophthalmia neonatorum 20
Opioid substitution therapy 69
Opportunistic fungal infection 3, 40, 43
Opportunistic neoplasms 44
OraQuick In-Home HIV testing kit 83
OraSure Technologies 83
Oropharyngeal candidiasis 43, 44
Oropharynx, disorders of 44
Outer membrane protein, major 60

P

Palindromic repeats, short 84
Papulopruritic eruption 36
Papulopruritic itch 35
Parasites 4
Pelvic inflammatory disease 5, 17, 20, 56
Pelvic pain, chronic 60
Penile
  cancer 41f
  discharge 22f
  shaft 9
Perinuclear draped 21f
Periurethral abscess 20
Pharyngeal gonorrhea 20
Podophyllin 29
Podophyllotoxin 28
Point-of-care 84
  dual testing method 82
Polymerase chain reaction 27

Polymorphic membrane proteins 60
Postpartum endometritis 16
Posttraumatic stress disorder 51
Preterm
    birth 16
    labor 16
Primary Health Centers 6, 73
Procaine penicillin 12
Proctocolitis 40
Prophylactic vaccines 55
Prostatitis 20
ProTide approach 83
Psoriasis 35, 37
Public and private sector collaboration 67
Public health measures 10
Purified protein derivative 29

R

Radioimmunoassay 20
Rapid diagnostic test 75
Rapid plasma reagin 9, 75
Rectal gonorrhea 19
Red Ribbon Club 6
Replicative reticulate body 85
Reproductive complications 17
Reproductive tract infection 2, 6, 65
    services delivery 74*fc*
Respiratory infections 82
Ribonucleic acid, single-stranded 33
Rovafovir etalafenamide 84

S

Salpingitis 20
Sampoorna Suraksha Strategy 69
Scabies 35
    crusted 35
Scrotal swelling 3
    painful 23
Seborrheic dermatitis 35, 36, 36*f*
Secnidazole 5
Seminal vesiculitis 20
Sex partners, management of 16, 17
Sex with men 47
Sex workers, female 70
Sexual abuse 47
    management of child with 52*b*
Sexual contact 9
Sexual health test 85
Sexual offences, protection of children 52
Sexually transmitted diseases 16
    management of 5, 82

Sexually transmitted infections 1, 3, 4, 6, 24, 38, 47, 48, 55, 65, 74*fc*, 76, 77*fc*, 82
    etiological classification of 4*t*
    in males and females, prevalence of 3*t*
    in sex with men population 48*b*
    incidence of 2*f*
    laboratory network 79*f*
    newer 47, 48
    syndromic management of 5*t*
    vaccines in 56*t*
Sexually transmitted infections control program 4, 65
    basic principles of 6*b*
Shigella
    flexneri 48
    reinfection cycle of 48
Silicone vaginal ring 83
Sinecatechins 28
Soft tissue infection 44
Staphylococcal infections 35
Staphylococcus
    aureus 44
    saprophyticus 18
Stevens–Johnson syndrome 18
Stigma, experience of 67
Strawberry cervix 16
Streptococci 14
Streptococcus pneumoniae 18
Subdermal implants 84
Sulfamethoxazole 11
Suraksha clinic 6
Surgical scissor excision 30
Swab tests 18
Syphilis 1, 3, 9, 38, 55, 56, 74, 82
    congenital 9
    early 12
    health check treponemal antibody test 83
    late 12
    primary 8, 9
    reverse
        testing for 75*f*
        treatment for 76*fc*
    secondary 9
    treatment of 12*t*
    vaccine, development of 58

T

T cells, resident memory 60
Tampons and intrauterine contraceptive device 14
Targeted syndrome 78
Telemedicine services 82

Tenofovir, toxicity of 84
Tenosynovitis 20
Tinidazole 21, 86
Tissue damage 19
TonB-dependent transporters 85
Tp0751 58
Transgender MSM 47
Treponema pallidum 8, 39, 47, 56, 58
    hemagglutination assay 75, 76
    particle agglutination 75, 76
Treponemal antibody testing 75*f*
Trichloroacetic acid solution 29
Trichomonas 1
    vaginalis 3, 16, 18, 21, 22*f*, 39, 56, 59, 86
        detection 85
Trichomoniasis 16, 17*t*, 40, 55, 56
Trimethoprim 11
Tritrichomonas foetus 59
Tumors
    benign 31
    malignant 31

U

Ulcerative lesions 1
Ureaplasma urealyticum 18, 21
Urethral discharge 18, 19*f*, 23, 23*t*
    syndrome 39
Urethral stricture 18
Urethritis 21
Urogenital system 18
Urogenital tract abscesses 56

V

Vaccine
    candidates 59-61
    development 57, 58
    need for 57, 58

Vaginal candidiasis 35
Vaginal culture 17
Vaginal discharge 23, 23*t*
    abnormal 14, 15*f*, 15*fc*
    infective causes 18*f*
    normal 14
    syndrome 5, 39
Vaginal flora
    healthy 14
    normal 14
Vaginal mucosa 39
Vaginitis 5
Valaciclovir 12
Valency 57
Varicella-zoster virus 42
Venereal disease research laboratory 38, 75
Virology 33
Viruses 4
Vulvovaginal candidiasis 17, 43

W

Walrinvax 57
Warts 35
Whiff test 16, 14
Whole genome sequencing 85
Wound infections 44

X

Xerosis 35

Y

Youth-focused programming 69

Z

Zika virus 48, 50